THE ROLE OF COMPANION ANIMALS IN COUNSELING AND PSYCHOLOGY

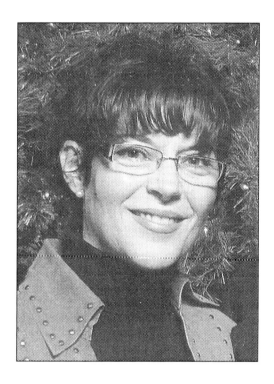

ABOUT THE AUTHOR

Jane K. Wilkes, R.N., M.A.P.P.C., has studied and worked within the fields of nursing, pastoral care, psychology, and counseling for 30 years. She is certified in Trauma Recovery and Animal-Assisted Therapy. Jane's Australian Labradoodle, Willy, has also been certified to work in Animal-Assisted Therapy. Jane's interests are focused on the implementation and promotion of animal-assisted therapy in all facets of mental health. Jane Wilkes is a member of the College and Association of Registered Nurses of Alberta, and the Alberta Association of Registered Nurses in Private Practice. She holds a master's degree in Counseling and Psychology and is a term instructor in the Psychiatric Nursing Program within the Faculty of Health and Community Studies at Grant MacEwan College in Edmonton, Alberta, Canada.

THE ROLE OF COMPANION ANIMALS IN COUNSELING AND PSYCHOLOGY

Discovering Their Use in the Therapeutic Process

By

JANE K. WILKES, R.N., M.A.P.P.C.

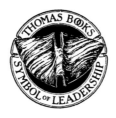

CHARLES C THOMAS • PUBLISHER, LTD.
Springfield • Illinois • U.S.A.

Published and Distributed Throughout the World by

CHARLES C THOMAS • PUBLISHER, LTD.
2600 South First Street
Springfield, Illinois 62704

This book is protected by copyright. No part of
it may be reproduced in any manner without written
permission from the publisher. All rights reserved.

© 2009 by CHARLES C THOMAS • PUBLISHER, LTD.

ISBN 978-0-398-07863-8 (paper)

Library of Congress Catalog Card Number: 2008048228

With THOMAS BOOKS *careful attention is given to all details of manufacturing
and design. It is the Publisher's desire to present books that are satisfactory as to their
physical qualities and artistic possibilities and appropriate for their particular use.*
THOMAS BOOKS *will be true to those laws of quality that assure a good name
and good will.*

*Printed in the United States of America
LAH-R-3*

Library of Congress Cataloging-in-Publication Data

Wilkes, Jane K.
 The role of companion animals in counseling and psychology : discovering
their use in the therapeutic process / by Jane K. Wilkes.
   p. cm.
 Includes bibliographical references and index.
 ISBN 978-0-398-07863-8 (pbk.)
 1. Pets--Therapeutic use. 2. Domestic animals--Therapeutic use. I. Title.

 RC489.P47W55 2009
 616.89'165--dc22

                                        2008048228

*In gratitude to canine companions,
who give so much, yet ask so little.
Simply put, they make the world
a better place.*

PREFACE

The human health benefits derived from relationships with companion animals have attracted a lot of scientific interest and research. However, there is a need for theoretical conceptualizations in order to understand the healing benefits of human-animal interactions. This book represents the author's journey into seeking out the answers to "how" and "why" companion animals play a role in counseling and psychology. It begins by describing how aspects of her personal story became integrated with current literature to guide the questions that became the focus of her master's thesis, which is the foundation of this publication.

The purpose of the project encompassed within this book was two-fold. The first goal was to discover the role of companion animals in the therapeutic process of counseling and psychology. In-depth semi-structured interviews were conducted with three psychologist participants who use animals in their therapy settings. The focus of the interviews was to determine their experiences of having a companion animal present during therapy sessions. The results revealed that pets in therapy: (1) *enhanced the therapeutic alliance/relationship*, (2) *enhanced the therapeutic environment*, (3) *enhanced professional practice*, and (4) *created a sense of sacredness*.

The second purpose of this book was to apply the four themes that arose from the interviews to Winnicott's concepts of the holding environment and transitional phenomena (Phillips, 1988). The results suggested that the therapy animals supplied qualities of the phenomena of "good-enough-mother," and in doing so, played a role in the creation and maintenance of what Winnicott referred to as "the holding environment." The therapy animals seemed to provide the trust and safety needed for clients to work within the transitional space and that the animals may act as transitional objects for some clients.

This book suggests that the therapy animals were extremely helpful in providing a sense of safety for traumatized clients and could act as catalysts, especially with defensive and/or detached clients. These conclusions appear to agree with Fine and Mio, who stated, "with the sensitive use of animals, [therapists] may very well achieve a therapeutic breakthrough" (2006, p. 514). It would seem that skilled therapists may find animal-assisted therapy to be a powerful tool to have at their disposal.

J.K.W.

ACKNOWLEDGMENTS

First and foremost, I would like to thank my husband, Brian, and children, Lindsey and Matthew, for their constant support, encouragement, and patience. Their belief in my abilities carried me through the rough patches and sustained me in moments of my own disbelief. I am truly blessed to have such a loving and wonderful family. Secondly, I would like to thank Dr. Margaret Clark, whose belief in my abilities and goodness allowed me to manifest a belief in myself.

I would like to thank Dennis Anderson, the director of The Chimo Project, for his support of the research project contained within this book. I would especially like to thank Kristine Anderson, the program manager of The Chimo Project, for her constant support and interest. I would also like to thank Dr. Jane Simington for her guidance in the completion of my thesis project which is the foundation of this book.

It has been said that there is nothing but heaven itself that is better than a friend who is truly a friend. I am blessed to have a friend such as this in Colleen Burrows. I thank her for serving as a constant cheerleader who called regularly to check up on my progress. She always managed to "prop me up" when I was feeling overwhelmed.

Lastly, I would like to thank my two dogs, Willy and Maggie, for being at my side day in and day out. Their "presence" supported me so many times when I began to falter. Through an encouraging paw, or a lick, or a nudge, my fears and frustrations would begin to dissipate. Their constant unconditional love served to remind me of why I was doing this thesis project in the first place.

CONTENTS

	Page
Preface	vii

Chapter 1. PICKING UP THE SCENT ... 3

Chapter 2. FOLLOWING THE TRAIL ... 19
Domestication of Companion Animals ... 19
The Biophilia Hypothesis ... 21
Research into the Human-Animal Bond ... 26
Social and Psychological Support Theory ... 29
From the Human-Animal Bond to Animal-Assisted Therapy ... 31

Chapter 3. UNEARTHING THE TREASURE ... 38
The Interview Questions ... 38
Need for the Project ... 39
Description of the Methods Used ... 39
Ethical Considerations ... 41
Collection of Information ... 42
Analysis and Interpretation of Interviews ... 51
Trustworthiness of Results ... 55

Chapter 4. ANALYZING THE FIND ... 56
Theme I: Enhanced Therapeutic Alliance/Relationship ... 56
Theme II: Enhanced Therapeutic Environment ... 61
Theme III: Enhanced Professional Practice ... 68
Theme IV: Creating a Sense of Sacredness ... 73

Chapter 5: GNAWING ON THE RAWHIDE ... 76
Description of Object Relations Theory and Winnicott's Concepts ... 76

xii   *The Role of Companion Animals in Counseling and Psychology*

Application of Themes to Winnicott's "Holding Environment" 79
Application of Themes to Winnicott's Transitional Phenomena 89
Conclusion 94

Chapter 6: SAVORING AND SHARING THE
        TREASURED FIND. 98
Implications for the Practice of Counseling and Psychology 98
Suggestions for Future Research. 104
Professional and Ethical Considerations 108
Conclusions 112

APPENDICES
A: Definition of Terms. 117
B: Interview Checklist. 121
C: Agreement To Be Interviewed 122
D: Agreement To Be Audiotaped. 124
E: Perspectives and Demographics 125
F: Transcriber's Agreement of Confidentiality. 127
G: Agreement of Confidentiality for Independent Judge 128
H: Delineating Units of Meaning. 129
I: Clustering Units of Meaning. 130
J: Themes. 132
K: Final Themes 135

Bibliography. 139
Index 153

THE ROLE OF COMPANION ANIMALS IN COUNSELING AND PSYCHOLOGY

Chapter 1

PICKING UP THE SCENT

During the aftermath of Hurricane Katrina in 2005, emergency efforts were difficult at best. In one particular situation, such efforts became almost impossible because a crying elderly woman needed to cling to her Yorkshire terrier dog as emergency workers attempted to lift her into an already overloaded helicopter. In his frustration, the attending trooper ordered, "You can't bring that." The older woman's desperate cries and pleas alerted the attending flight surgeon. The trooper's reluctant response to the flight surgeon's request for the dog was accompanied by "Sir, we have orders not to bring on any dogs." The surgeon's response was quick and effective. "That's not a dog–that's medicine" (Ubelacker, 2005, p. A2).

This story reflects two distinct aspects of this book. First, it speaks to my experience of desperately clinging to a furry friend when feeling frightened and confused. Second, the flight surgeon's comment that the dog was medicine echoes my belief, cultivated through actually experiencing the healing capabilities of canine companions. Through this experience, a review of the literature, and the discoveries to be presented in this book, I have come to acknowledge that companion animals provide the perfect mirror into our darkness while providing the unconditional love and acceptance needed to venture into unknown territory. Although dogs, as companions and helpers, will be the major focus of this writing, I now conclude that all animals have a way of linking us to something deep within, something that touches us intensely, something that makes a connection to our hearts and to our souls.

Many people look back on their relationships with pets with a fondness hard to put into words. They see their animals as significant others who have served as important markers to the various transitions and phases of their lives (Jalongo, 2004). I know that my dogs played a large role in helping me survive the difficult years of childhood. I often wonder if I would be here today had I not had the constant love of my faithful canine companions to keep me from putting an end to my suffering.

Throughout my childhood, and indeed to this day, my dogs have been there as a source of support and love. My broken childhood was one of loneliness and fear. As a young child, I dealt with the trauma of witnessing and being pulled into my parents' violent fights, as well as the daily grind of living in a home filled with anger and tension. The worst part of my wounding stemmed from my mother's deep resentment toward me. For some strange reason, she viewed me as some sort of competition. In later years, I came to understand that she did not see me as her daughter, but as the other woman vying for the attention of her man.

My mother's resentment of me was demonstrated recently. My brothers took over her estate following her diagnosis of Alzheimer's and needed my okay to sell a piece of property held within my mother's estate. In order to explain why, my eldest brother showed me my mother's will, and, although I was not surprised, I was saddened to see that she continued to see me as competition even after my father's death. When listing the beneficiaries of her estate, she gave a reason for not considering me as equal to my brothers. She wrote, "Because of the gifts bestowed upon Jane by her father. . . ." My father never left me any material gifts, but I guess his love for me was too much for my mother to handle even after he was gone.

I spent years trying to win my mother's approval and to gain an understanding of why I carried such profound pain. To be seen as unworthy by your own mother leaves a hole in your soul that aches beyond belief. The mental and physical abuse I endured from my mother's inability to face whatever it was she projected onto me left me confused and anxious. There were many times that I found life unbearable, and it was at those times that my little dog literally kept me from the action of suicide.

I remember one incident in particular during a time when the urge to shut off the pain began to take a firm hold. That day, my mother's attack on my character had been particularly venomous. My two older brothers joined in, seeming to find a sense of joy in helping to destroy what little self-esteem remained. Once the supper dishes were done, I went to my room. No one noticed that I had taken a paring knife with me. I stared at the knife as I wept silently on my bed, filled with a sense of hopelessness. I soon heard a scratching on my door accompanied with anxious yipping and whining. I opened the door to my room and Scamper, my dog, began jumping up on me. As I knelt on the floor to pick him up, I began to sob. In my brokenness, my little furry friend brought healing. His wet kisses helped to heal my most profound inner worries and fears. Through a long cuddle with him, I felt I could once again face the human world.

One may ask where my father was in all of this. I believe my dad truly loved me; however, having to deal with my extremely moody and needy mother day in and day out left him with little energy for a relationship with me. My father should have shielded me from my mother's abuse, but he did not and probably could not. For many years, I managed to excuse and rationalize my father's failure to protect by attributing it to my own unworthiness in order to preserve the bond I had with him. I placed my father on a pedestal and attempted to meet the high demands he placed on me by becoming a high achiever who demanded personal perfection.

Most of the nurturing I received as a child came from the family dogs. Our first little dog, Scamper, carried me through to my high school years. He helped me cope with the sadness that goes along with feeling unwanted. The rejection I experienced resulted in a profound sense of isolation. Upon reflection, I realize that although I felt disconnected to humankind in my early years, I was blessed to have been able to acquire a sense of connection from my dog. Scamper's unconditional love provided the hope of a better tomorrow. His caring eyes allowed me to gain inklings of self-worth.

When Scamper died, I was devastated. I came home after school in mid-September to find a note on the kitchen table that said, "Scamper died. We've gone to bury him." My marks soon began to fall, and I felt a heavy cloak of depression descend upon me. Life at home was a nightmare, and I had no ally to turn to when I felt the chaotic emotions begin to overwhelm me.

In November, my girlfriend's dog had puppies, and I managed to receive permission from my parents to keep a cute little black bundle of fur. It was not an easy task, but I seemed to intuitively know that I needed a dog to nurture and support me through the remaining years in the family home. Benji soon became my port in the storm.

Winnicott believed "There is no health for the human being who has not been started off well enough by the mother" (Winnicott, 2005, p. 15). In my own experience, feeling unwanted left me catering to the needs of others, and the internal object of my mother became the critic that lived within my psyche. The abuse and trauma I endured caused me to become hypervigilant, and the constant sense of foreboding left me exhausted. Restful sleep was difficult to achieve. Yet on the nights I was able to have my little dog sleep beside me, I was able to have a peaceful rest. I was soothed by the notion my furry companion could take over, ever alert to any sound or motion that could mean danger.

My dog acted as a sentinel, and I felt protected from the demons that haunted me and the humans that could hurt me. If I woke during the night, I would reach out to ensure my furry avenger remained at my side. He would respond to my touch with a gentle lick, which served to communicate all was well. Scamper did what my mother could not; he assured me that I safe and that I was worthy of guardianship. My dogs were a Godsend, and I was supplied with comfort and warmth in my aloneness.

The dogs with which I had been gifted throughout my childhood served to meet many of my otherwise unmet needs in situations in which I found myself unable to trust a fellow human being. They made me feel that I was "okay" through their unrestricted approval, and absolute devotion. They were my confidantes and my caregivers. When in doubt, I could ask my canine companions questions, and the answer was often found in the soulful expressions I received from their friendly faces. I experienced a sense of redemption in myself by relating my greatest fears into the warm, soft ear of my soul friends, for they allowed me to express my uncertainties about myself without the fear of rejection.

The pets in my childhood gave me what my parents could not—unconditional love, acceptance, and a sense of belonging. My dogs have walked beside me throughout my life and continue to journey with me as companions as I work toward healing the pain of my past. To this very day, my dogs are my best friends. They are medicine; they enrich and enhance my mental, physical, psychological, and spiritual health simply by their presence.

I had never realized how important the role my animals played in my childhood was until I took a course in child and adolescent psychology and counseling. After coming to fully appreciate the nurturing needed to ensure healthy growth and development, I began to wonder how on earth I made it out of my childhood home without some severe psychological disorder. Studying Bowlby's (1989) theory of attachment behavior, I was struck with a curiosity as to how I had developed the ability to "attach" in any functional manner when I had never been supplied with what Bowlby believed necessary for mental health. He felt secure attachment depended on a child's experiencing a "warm, intimate, and continuous relationship" with a primary caregiver. The relationship I had with my primary caregiver was anything but warm, intimate and continuous.

Bowlby (1988) believed that children need to know "for sure" that, no matter what happens, they have a welcoming home where they will be "nourished physically and emotionally, comforted if distressed, reassured if frightened" (Bowlby, 1988, p. 11). I have no memories of running home to be comforted in the warm and protective arms of a loving caregiver. In fact, I dreaded going home. I would do whatever I could to stay away as long as possible. As I got older, I won many service awards for my extracurricular volunteer work. Unbeknown to the teachers at my school and the church leaders in my Catholic community of faith, they actually provided me with a service–they gave me a legitimate excuse to stay away from home.

No, I did not have a welcoming home but what I did have was an animal that was always there to offer affection, intimacy, and unconditional love. I was deeply attached to the dogs in my life. During this course it dawned on me that it was through my connection to my dogs that I was able to acquire the skills needed for attachment to people. The connection between me and my animals formed a bridge that allowed communication with my core. This core contains spirit, and it is spirit that links all people to each other and the world around them. I now recognize that because I did not have other people, my dogs supplied the link necessary for me to connect to the world around me. In doing so, they supplied the essential ingredients to sustain and enhance my mental and spiritual health.

Recognizing that my animals had played a significant role in my growth and development led me to explore literature related to the human-animal bond. I was drawn to the work of Kidd and Kidd

(1985), whose studies indicated that children are able to gain support from their pets when they are distressed and experiencing feelings of fear, loneliness, and rejection, and to the work of Bachman and Bachman (2003), who believed that pets often provide protective factors by meeting the emotional needs of children who are abused and neglected. They suggest that these protective factors can assist children to develop psychological health by providing a sense of security when they are dealing with difficult emotions. It seems that pets often serve as silent counselors, best friends, and even surrogate siblings (Arehart-Treichel, 1982; Beck & Katcher, 1996; Brown, Richards & Wilson, 1996).

Studies on high-school students have shown pet ownership may be beneficial to both adolescents who are having challenges in personal independence and those with mature interfamilial relationships (Davis, 1987; Fine, 2000; Kidd & Kidd, 1990). Pets play a particularly important role in the lives of children who have inadequate or destructive family and social environments (Blue, 1986; Levinson, 1971; Robin, tenBensel, Quingly & Anderson, 1983). This was certainly true in my experience.

As I reached adolescence, my mother's resentment of me seemed to grow. It was as if the onset of puberty triggered an increase in her sense of my posing a threat as the other woman in the house. Thus, while I struggled through the normal difficulties inherent in a teenager's life, I also dealt with more frequent and malicious attacks on my character. During this time, my dogs were an anchor, providing a steady, reliable source of affection in a life filled with insecurity and pain.

Dogs have a history as scavengers (Nicoll, 2005; Sams & Carson, 1999). Because of this, my canine companions were able to dig deep through the rubbish of my inner world and help me find the kernel of truth hidden away behind a façade of control. They were able to assist me in finding some sense of truth about who I was in all the chaos and were able to connect with me spiritually by reading my body language and smelling my feelings of confusion and fear. My dogs experienced and anticipated my physical and inner pains. Their abilities to accept me as my naked authentic self brought comfort as they guided me down the road to self-discovery.

In gaining insight into the profound positive effect my animals had on my well being, I developed a deep appreciation for the love and nurturing they had provided. I soon began to wonder about the possibilities for healing that companion animals could bring to children within the environment of counseling and psychology. I received permission from my instructor to pursue this further through writing my final paper in child and adolescent psychology and counseling on pet-assisted therapy.

Completing this book required an in-depth exploration of the research on the relationships between animals and children. The deeper I delved into this literature, the more I awakened memories of my own difficult childhood and of the numerous positive and even life-saving experiences I had with my dogs. As the memories flooded and the images surfaced, I recognized how frequently I had witnessed traumatic events as a child and how deeply traumatized I had been. According Jon to Allen, "Ideally, parenting is the essential buffer against trauma. Yet parenting can fail to buffer trauma and, at worst, it can itself be a source of trauma" (1995, p. 37). It seems I was one of those unfortunate children traumatized by those who were supposed to love and protect me. Along with "the more cumulative traumas of unmet dependency needs" (Kalsched, 2005, p. 1), I had witnessed and experienced the terror of physical and mental abuse.

Trauma causes uncontrollable hyperarousal from an upset in physiological regulation, so a child needs to have some means to regain a sense of security (Allen, 1995). As I pondered this, I remembered all the times I clung to my little dog for dear life during terrifying moments in my younger years. Often, I would hide away in my secret spots, feeling confused, alone, and full of anxiety and fear. It seemed my little dog would always find me as if coming to my rescue. I would hang on to him tightly finding comfort in his cool wet nose as he gently licked the tears from my face. I saw a profound caring in his big brown eyes and was reassured through his warm, furry body.

I believe the unconditional love I felt during these times of turmoil was not from my furry friend alone. I believe that the loving presence of a Higher Power used my little animal as a vehicle to bring the support and comfort I needed. Scamper kept me connected to this divine power in moments of utter terror. He kept me connected to life, and in doing so, he kept me connected to spirit.

Through my little dog, I learned the skills needed to calm myself. He taught me how to ground myself in the midst of chaos and how to experience the love of another being as comfort and reassurance. I guess he actually provided me with the teaching I needed in order to learn how to self-soothe. Strand's (2004) research suggested that companion animals help children cope with traumatic events through physiologically relaxing the child, so it would seem my thoughts are correct.

I continued to study the concept of animal-assisted therapy well after my term paper had been completed. Then, while taking courses in life span psychology and the individual theories of counseling and psychology, I became interested in the work of Winnicott (1896-1971). It seemed his concept of transitional objects (1953) was reminiscent of the safety and security I had received from my dog. The transitional object represents the first "not-me possession" and is the child's first use of a symbol and the first experience of creativity or play. It is an object chosen by the child and is usually in the form of a blanket or teddy bear. This object provides the child with the safety needed in order to let go and begin to separate from the symbiotic relationship with his or her mother and develop a more independent existence.

I eventually found a study by Triebenbacher (1998), in which she looked at pets as transitional objects in children's emotional development. Her results indicated that pets do serve functions similar to those offered by inanimate transitional objects. There were also other authors who suggested that companion animals could be viewed as a higher form of transitional object for adults as well as children (Bridger, 1970; Perin, 1981; Serpell, 1993).

Aaron Katcher (2000), a psychiatrist and professor at the University of Pennsylvania, felt the context of Winnicott's concept of transitional relationship and transitional object could be used as a means to understand the relationship between pets and people. He suggested the animals act as, and be referred to as, transitional beings. Unlike inanimate transitional objects such as a stuffed toys or blankets, a transitional being moves and shows intentional behavior that is more like a person. Importantly, they can never contradict the attributes projected onto them with words. He writes, "Animals make good transitional beings. . . . Throughout our entire lives, our animals are there as transitional objects, being what we imagine them to be, serving as vehicles for projecting those admirable traits that we find so lacking in fellow human beings" (pp. 468–469).

As I began to further grasp an understanding into Winnicott's views on healthy development and the concept of transitional phenomena, I connected my experience of being nurtured by my dog to the characterization of "good-enough-mother." Kahane defines this phenomenon as "a protectively hovering spirit who, always striving to adapt to her infant's needs, provides a holding environment in which the infant is contained" (1993, pp. 278–279). For as far back as I can remember, my protective little dog was always present, helping to contain the overwhelming emotions of my inner world as I worked to understand them in relation to the reality of my outer world.

According to Kahane (1993), Winnicott's twofold formulations of transitional phenomena act as agents of the good-enough-mother. The first is that of transitional object, and, as stated earlier, it has been suggested that pets can fill this role. The second phenomenon is the transitional space, which can be defined as that intermediate area between the subjective and the objective. This space involves creativity and is where Winnicott believed positive growth occurred.

The transitional space lies between reality and nonreality and is where children and adults risk, explore, and discover. It connects the conscious to the unconscious, and animals have been known to act as mediators to the unconscious (Serpell, 2000b). While reading through the literature on animal-assisted therapy in the realm of counseling and psychology, I discovered that many therapists have noticed that pets can act as a catalyst in enabling clients to reveal difficult thoughts, feelings, and conflicts arising from their inner world (Mason & Hagan, 1999; Reichert, 1998; Wells, Rosen & Walshaw, 1997). It would seem that as mediators of the unconscious, animals could promote opportunities for growth by enhancing opportunities within the transitional space.

Having come to the conclusion that companion animals have the attributes included in the concept of the good-enough-mother, my curiosity arose as to whether a devoted and loving companion animal could assist in the creation and maintenance of what Winnicott (1965) coined the holding environment during therapy sessions. The term "holding environment" has to do with psychologically framing, holding, and contextualizing clients in such a way that they feel validated, encouraged, and supported (Phillips, 1988).

Winnicott's direct observation of mothers and babies, along with collecting careful histories, provided him with the understanding that "most mothers provide their infants with an emotionally healthy environment" (Wyatt-Brown, 1993, p. 293). He also came to understand that mothers held an innate desire to meet their infant's needs, to become the "ordinary good mother" who creates "a good-enough environment" for her child to develop and grow (Winnicott, 1949, p. 245). It is from these realizations that Winnicott formulated what came to be known as the holding environment. For Winnicott (1987), and those who were influenced by his work, a therapist's first and foremost responsibility was "the provision of a congenial milieu, a 'holding environment' analogous to maternal care" (Phillips, 1988, p. 11).

Winnicott (1958) suggested that the backdrop for the development of a capacity to be alone was formed through the child's experience of being alone in the mother's presence. Winnicott's notion of aloneness in the mother's presence also represents a metaphor for an essential element of the holding environment within the psychotherapeutic process. Slochower (1996) states, "For those people who have sufficiently internalized a sense of whole aloneness, the [therapeutic] setting itself may create a space within which such aloneness may productively be used. However, for those individuals whose sense of self is especially vulnerable to external assault, a therapeutic holding process around self-involvement may become pivotal" (p. 62).

In Winnicott's view, there were people who had experienced such severe failure of the early holding environment that they lived with the feeling they had not yet started to exist. "Their lives were characterized by a sense of futility born of compliance" (Phillips, 1988, p. 127). For these clients, it was imperative to provide a therapeutic milieu conducive to holding in order to restore the environment of early infancy, where the mothering should have facilitated the processes of integration, personalization and realization.

In providing structure and a consistent venue for the client, it is believed that a sense of safety and trust will develop from the "holding" experience. The holding environment sets the stage for the client to experience feelings and work through conflicts while the therapist "contains" overwhelming emotions. This act of containing is crucial and enables the client to resolve issues without the therapist's having to anxiously look for a cure (Winnicott, 1964).

I believe it was through the holding environment provided by my companion animals that I found a way to preserve a sense of trust in what was untrustworthy, safety in situations that were unsafe, control in situations that were terrifying and unpredictable, and power in a situation in which I was helpless. In essence, my dogs provided me with the nurturing experience of the good-enough-mother.

Picking Up the Scent 13

Dealing with the trauma of my past has not been an easy journey. The wounding I received was deep, and the scars are many. However, I believe I would have been unable to remain psychologically intact without the interventions of my dogs. They played a significant role in my growth and development. Scamper and Benji entered my life as trusted daily companions, and they were an unexpected spiritual presence that entered at moments of vulnerability, when I was open to their profound teachings.

The anthropologist Loren Eiseley said, "One does not meet oneself until one catches the reflection from an eye other than human" (as cited in Lasher, 1996, p. 5). Eiseley was not referring to the ordinary self of everyday reality, but the self that composes our inner core and provides us with the sense of aliveness spoken of by Winnicott–the part of our being that connects and vibrates with all other senses (Phillips, 1988). My pets allowed for the provision of an environment in which I was able to enter into my own center and listen to the stirrings of my own soul. In doing so, I connected to the spirit and came to know that being alive means loving, and being loved.

On the fringe of most spiritual traditions is the belief that humans have a spiritual connection to animals and animal spirits. For most of human history, animals have occupied a central position in theories concerning spirituality and the treatment of sickness and disease. Greek mythology tells the story of the centaur, Chiron, who was half-man half-horse. As the first physician, and the teacher of Aesculapius (sometimes referred to as Asklepios), he could be considered the first pet therapist (Beck & Katcher, 1996). Aesculapius was known as the god of medicine and as the divine physician. It is said that he employed dogs, who were believed to carry the power of the god and able to cure illness with licks from their tongues (Schoen, 2001; Serpell, 2006).

In ancient Egypt, the jackal-headed Anubis served as protector (Sams & Carson, 1999) and physician to gods (Schoen, 2001). The Egyptians also worshiped the goddess Bast, who was often depicted either as a cat or with a cat's head. In Scandinavian lore, the cat was associated with Freyja, the goddess of fertility. Shasthi, the Hindu goddess of fertility, is depicted riding a cat (Andrews, 2003).

During the early centuries of Christianity, traces of the animist belief of ancient shamanic ideas and practices, which involved the supernatural power of animal and animal spirits, were still prevalent throughout Europe. In addition to being healers, "Most of the early Celtic saints and holy men of Britain and Ireland were distinguished by their special rapport with animals, and many, according to legend, experienced bodily transformation into animal form" (Serpell, 2006, p. 9).

St. Francis of Assisi, who appears to have been influenced by Irish monastic traditions, was described as a "nature mystic." Among many other wondrous deeds, he was known to preach sermons to rapt audiences of birds and was noted for being able to pacify rabid wolves (Armstrong, 1973 as cited in Serpell, 2006). "St. Roch, who, like Aesculapius, was generally depicted in the company of a dog, seems to have been cured of plague sores by the licking of his canine companions" (Serpell, 2006, p. 10). St. Bernard, St. Christopher, and a number of other saints were associated with dogs and believed to be healers.

In the shamanic tradition, animals are placed at the center of awareness. Among many shamanic cultures, a child is given an animal spirit as a vision and a name. The child, growing up with this identification, can call on the animal's special energies and strengths; the child's spirit and the animal's spirit are considered one (Lasher, 1996). The idea that children have an inherent fascination with and affection for animals is held within all cultures. In western culture, children are identified with animals through the telling of stories and making of television programs that are based on various animal characters. We also provide children with stuffed animals on the assumption they will form a bond with these cuddly representations of the animal kingdom (Loar & Colman, 2004; Melson, 2001).

Lasher (1996), a psychologist who specializes in relational theory, studied shamanism and Taoism. She believed that Western culture's use of animal metaphor and story with children is actually our way of teaching them about animal spirits. She also believed that when we choose to make any animal part of our lives, we are in essence doing something quite similar to the ancient practice of the shaman who calls upon the animal spirits for assistance. "Like shamans, we turn to animals for some needed insight or healing" (1996, p. 11).

Lasher (1996) believed that, although we do not have the level of training and awareness of a shaman, we may stumble upon an animal, "seemingly by accident," that brings us the energy we need at the time. This is the animal medicine spoken of in many aboriginal cultures. We connect to the spirit of the animal in such a way as to renew our own inner spirit and learn an important teaching. Through this connection to the animal, we may become aware of some aspect of the self that has been lost, unacknowledged, or partly blocked by the pressures of human society. We reconnect to the core of ourselves by following an instinct that, in spite of our complex and sometimes insane civilization, has never been lost.

Perhaps the dogs in my childhood, and indeed throughout my life, brought me the animal medicine I needed to heal. Dogs represent the power of loyalty to self and self-truths. The medicine of dog embodies the loving gentleness of best friend and the half-wild protector energy of territorial imperative (Sams & Carson, 1999). Through my connection to my dogs, I was able to call upon a power greater than my own to become a survivor rather than a victim. I believe that dogs absorb our many projections in their wanting to do anything to serve us. As stated by Sams and Carson in the book *Medicine Cards*, "Dog has been considered the servant of humanity throughout history. . . . Canines are genuinely service-orientated animals" (1999, p. 93). A dog honors its gifts and is loyal to the trust placed in its care.

In shamanic tradition, the spirits of animals contain lessons for deeper understanding of self, other, and the universe around us. Perhaps like the shaman, I entered the world of my canine companions, who acted as guides, leading me toward developing a deeper understanding of life. My love for my dogs led me on a path of soul discovery simply by being present to the "now."

In watching my animals take joy in the newly fallen snow, leap over bushes while chasing a butterfly, or roll happily in the cool grass on a hot day, I felt connected to something bigger. My pets were always ready to share the wonders they saw in the world, yet could also be ferocious in their protection of me if they sensed a threat. They have shown me more compassion than I would have thought any being was capable of showing. Most of all, my dogs have provided much of the nurturing I needed to build a fairly healthy psychological structure. My furry friends were my good-enough-mothers until I could be a good-enough-mother to myself. In reclaiming the "power of dog," I learned a loyalty to self and self-truths. I took on the "medicine of dog" and became my own best friend (Sams & Carson, 1999).

Although most of the research on animal-assisted therapy concerns the bond between dogs and humans, cats are also companion animals to many and have been used in therapeutic work. Cats have been observed as taking on the role of the other through contemplating the feelings and expectations of others and acting according to their perceptions (Alger & Alger, 2003). Cats are at home in the dark and symbolize magic, mystery, and independence (Andrews, 2003). It would seem that cats are also mediators to the unconscious.

The idealized love of my dogs had little room for competition or comparison. In viewing my pets throughout the years as the protectively hovering spirits who adapted to my needs and provided a holding environment, I came to see how they could perhaps do the same for others (Kahane, 1993). As suggested by ethologist Konrad Lorenz (1952), dogs transfer their mother love onto us (as cited in Nicoll, 2005). Mother love is the perfected idealized love for which we all long. It is the complete submission to provide care and nurturance to someone. This devotional love is why I suggest that dogs, and perhaps cats, could play a role in the creation of a holding environment for clients. As stated by Nicoll, "Their natural ability to nurture surpasses many human attempts" (2005, p. 22).

During the process of taking my master's level of study, I began probing into the ugly secrets of my past so that I could begin to bind my own wounds. Nouwen stated, "Behind the dirty curtain of our painful symptoms there is something great to be seen" (1979, p. 44). As I cleaned out the dark corners and opened closed doors in order to heal, I took the wounds of my childhood and found a source of profound light.

I transformed expressions of despair into signs of hope for healing through animal-assisted therapy. My wounds and pains have become an opening for a new theoretical view of the role on animals in counseling and psychology. "Sometimes the greater part of genius is simply recognizing what is right in front of us" (Smith, as cited in Crawford & Pomerinke, 2003, p. 11). Nouwen stated, "Ministry can indeed be a witness to the living truth that the wound, which causes us to suffer now, will be revealed to us later as the place where God intimated his new creation" (1979, p. 96). Perhaps the suffering of my past was meant to steer me toward understanding the importance of the human-animal bond. In the writing of this book, I was called to be a wounded healer and share the gift of healing which I believe could be available when a companion animal is present in the therapeutic environment of counseling and psychology.

I have come to fully appreciate how my canine companions filled the role of good-enough-mother throughout my difficult childhood. They provided me with a holding environment in which I could feel safe enough to explore and grow. This knowledge made me wonder whether a companion animal could do the same for clients, especially those whose past hurts make trusting another human being difficult. I wondered if I could share the gifts I had received from my pets by exploring the possibility of companion animals doing much the same for clients by simply being "present" during therapy sessions. I asked myself, "Could the pets assisting the therapist create the safety and comfort needed to build a holding environment to provide a felt sense of security through filling the role of a protectively hovering spirit or good-enough-mother within the therapeutic arena?"

In order to explore my ponderings, I conducted an in-depth literature search and also conducted a phenomenological study. Participants were all registered psychologists who had experience working with and without a companion animal present in the room while they conducted therapy session with clients.

This book was guided by the question, *What is the companion animal's role within the therapeutic process of counseling and psychology?* This question would serve to help me discover what exactly it was that companion animals provided clients during counseling sessions but was not the question presented to participants. This was done to ensure their responses were in a pure form, not tainted by the word role. The question chosen to open the interview allowed for the essence of their experience to emerge from within.

The first question was, *What is your experience of having a companion animal present during sessions with clients?* This nondirected question was used in order to allow for a more holistic description. Participants discussed and reflected on this until the topic was exhausted. There was little interruption on my part, except to clarify or deepen the participants' responses. The interview was completed by asking the question, *What value, if any, has been derived from the presence of the companion animal?* This second question focused on aspects of the experience that were perceived as valuable in the therapeutic process of counseling and psychology.

Once the interviews were completed and transcribed, I analyzed the results and applied them to the contextual framework of object relations theory and Winnicott's concept of the good-enough-mother and holding environment. The discoveries documented in this book represent a means to further understand how companion animals may or may not assist counselors/psychologists within the psychotherapeutic process of counseling and psychology.

Chapter 2

FOLLOWING THE TRAIL

In 1855, Chief Seattle of the Duwamish Tribe wrote to the President of the United States asking, "What is man without beasts? If all the beasts are gone man would die from great loneliness of spirit, for whatever happens to the beasts also happens to man. All things are connected. Whatever befalls the earth, befalls the sons of the earth" (as cited in Fogle, 1981, p. 334).

DOMESTICATION OF COMPANION ANIMALS

Domestication of a species of animals occurs when "the care, feeding and, above all, the breeding of a species comes under the control of man" (Kretchmer & Fox, 1975, as cited in Messent & Serpell, 1981, p. 6). The worth of most domesticated animals is measured by the practical services and economic resources they provide.

The dog is generally thought to be the oldest of domestic animal species (Zeuner, 1963), with the earliest fossil remains from Iraq and Israel dating as far back as 12,000 years (Borowski, 1998; Davis & Valla, 1978). In the United States, finds have dated back about 10,000 years (Lawrence, 1967). Fossils in Denmark and the United Kingdom date back about 9,000 years (Musil, 1970) and from China about 7,000 years (Olsen & Olsen, 1977). Recent discoveries in China indicate there may have been a possible association between a "wolflike canid" and Peking man as early as 500,000 years ago (Messent & Serpell, 1981, p. 7).

When pondering the relationship between pets and people, a major question arises in regard to what social and/or environmental factors led to the switch from the mere capture and taming of wild animals to the process of true domestication. The possibility that dogs and cats were domesticated solely as items of food is supported by few authors (Messent & Serpell, 1981). Although the dog, unlike the cat, continues to be eaten in certain parts of the world such as the Far East and the Americas (Zeuner, 1963), this practice is definitely not widespread. It seems most likely that the practice of eating dogs originated as a temporary/starvation measure (Messent & Serpell, 1981).

The dog and cat were the first to achieve the status of domestic pets. This most likely resulted from changes in the climate of the Mesolithic period when societies moved toward a richer and more settled way of life. According to Messent and Serpell, "these species were able to transfer their normal social attachments to man and to behave toward him in a manner that was interpreted as friendly, affectionate, and companionable" (1981, p. 20). Over the years, the anthropomorphic and friendly qualities of dogs and cats have been enhanced through selective breeding, and this has, in turn, firmly cemented the bond between humans and companion animals.

In the last few decades, there has been a drastic change in attitude toward animals considered to act as companions for human beings. The term pet was first applied to the indulged, spoiled child. However, by the sixteenth century, the word had migrated to other small, childlike creatures such as cats, dogs, and young farm animals (Palmatier, 1995). The term companion animal became a popular alternative to the word pet in the 1990s. According to Irvine, "companion animals remain 'other' than human but in a sense worth honoring, rather than one of inferiority" (2004, p. 58).

Sarmicanic (2004) states the current use of the term "companion animal" as an alternative to pet emphasizes a change that has taken place in the way humans view domestication. There is now a marked difference between the relationship humans have with animals that have been domesticated for economic purposes and what they have with those that they choose to bring into their homes and their hearts. People use the term companion animal to denote the animals that are kept "primarily for social or emotional reasons rather than for economic purposes" (Serpell & Paul, 1994, p. 129). The difference between a domesticated animal and a companion animal is that the value of owning a companion animal is derived "from the relationship itself," rather than for reasons of practicality or economic benefit (Sarmicanic, 2004, p. 42).

THE BIOPHILIA HYPOTHESIS

In the nineteenth century, a few scientific studies looking at the human-animal bond began to appear in relation to the startling growth in the popularity of domestic pets. Most notable were the studies conducted by the renowned American psychologist Granville Stanley Hall, who in 1882 established an experimental psychology laboratory at Johns Hopkins University. Hall is the founder of child psychology and emphatically expounded his belief that ontogeny recapitulates phylogeny – "the development of an individual organism from embryo to adult duplicates the evolutionary development of the species" (Schoen, 2001, p. 50). Thus, as children mature, they replicate the development of our earliest forebears. Because of this, Hall believed that children should be surrounded by animals, "just as humankind was in the hunter/gatherer stage of its evolutionary past" (p. 50).

Hall's theories did not spur much research. However, Konrad Lorenz, who took a special interest in the relationship between humans and animals, alluded to the human longing for a bond with nature in his 1952 book *King Solomon's Ring*. He believed that humans' yearning for a connection with nature could be compared with the emotion involved in our longing for love and friendship (as cited in Hines, 2003, pp. 7–8).

It was not until the 1960s that serious study in the human-animal bond began. It was spurred on when psychologists observed changes in human behavior patterns due to animal companions. An example was Heiman (1965), who wrote about his observations that pets helped to maintain psychological equilibrium within psychoanalytic theory (Sable, 1995).

Many researchers were attempting to find a conceptual framework to use in understanding the human-animal bond. In 1984, biologist E. O. Wilson advanced Hall's earlier work in his conceptualization of the Biophilia Hypothesis (Wilson, 1984). He suggested that a predisposition to attune to animals and other living things is part of the human evolutionary heritage, a product of our coevolution as omnivores with animals and plants on which survival depend.

Biophilia is a unifying evolutionary concept coined by Wilson (Kellert & Wilson, 1993; Wilson, 1984). This hypothesis "posits that because humans co-evolved with animals in their natural settings, the survival of Homo sapiens fundamentally depended on alert and careful monitoring of animal and plant life" (Melson, 2000, p. 376). Animals became sentinels for human beings, with their behavior signifying both safety and danger. In other words, biophilia is a theoretical perspective that permits the study of people's interactions with animals or nature without making any assumptions about the way animals or trees or natural spaces are represented in the mind.

Wilson came to believe the human brain was structured to pay selective attention to other kinds of life, and, as a result, contact with other species, plant and animal, may have important influences on cognition, health, and well-being. The Biophilia Hypothesis suggests that animals are necessary to think and perceive (Kellert & Wilson, 1993; Wilson, 1984).

Wilson (1984, 1993) suggested that throughout most of human evolutionary development, fitness was increased by an ability to hunt animals and locate sources of vegetable food. Because of this, the brain was hardwired with a predisposition to pay attention to animals and the stimulus properties of the surrounding environment (Beck & Katcher, 2003).

According to many of those who believe in the Biophilia Hypothesis, we are genetically programmed to live in a symbiotic fashion with nature (Fogle, 1981; Newby, 1999). Our genetic evolution developed in such a way as to require that humans live in close relationship with the rest of creation. Fogle stated, "It is only in the last 20,000 years that we have hived ourselves off from our roots" (1981, p. 334).

The Biophilia Hypothesis and Human Health

Evidence appears to back up the Biophilia Hypothesis. In the 1960s and 1970s, there was a trend to build buildings without windows (Newby, 1999). "Alarm bells" went off when one researcher discovered that people in windowless postoperative intensive care units were twice more likely to be in a confused and hallucinogenic state than were patients with windows (Wilson, 1972). Ulrich (1984) also found that the wounds from a gallbladder operation healed, on average, a whole day earlier if the patients had a view of the park from their room. Seasonal affective disorder occurs because "artificial light does not trigger the same metabolic processes as natural light, and insufficient natural light can bring on confusion and depression" (Newby, 1999, p. 211). People seem to need to maintain a connection to nature.

Animal contact has been demonstrated to favorably influence the development of communication skills in young children (Filiatre, Millot & Montagner, 1983; Guttman, Predovic & Zemanek, 1983). Melson (2001) argues that many cultures elaborate on the natural attraction children have to animals. "Biophilia depicts children as born assuming a connection with other living things. The emotions and personalities of animals, real and symbolic, are immediate to children in the same way that the emotions and personalities of people are" (2001, p. 19).

This natural attraction to animals allows the animals to enter the drama of a child's life in direct and powerful ways. Since every human child begins life situated in what adults call the animal world, animals are readily accessed by children as material in the development of self. In his essay entitled "Totem and Taboo," Freud wrote that denying human bonds with animals "is still as foreign to the child as it is to the savage or to primitive man" (1913, p. 7) (as cited in Melson, 2001, p. 20).

The Biophilia Hypothesis and the Christian Bible

"The sign of the cross invites us to connect–to connect all that we value in life, to see in one pattern our deepest beliefs and experiences" (Eaton, 1995, p. ix). The Biophilia Hypothesis is about connecting with our evolutionary roots and our genetically programmed interrelationship with all of nature. The Bible speaks of the ideal of a loving community of all the species through creation stories. Man was fashioned like a clay figurine and then animated by a puff of the Lord's breath (Genesis, 2:4a–3:25).

The Bible goes on to tell of the delightful garden He prepared for the "Earth-man" to care for. But the Creator did not believe it was right for Man not to have a companion, so the Lord fashioned every kind of animal and bird and brought them to meet Man. "As each was brought the Man gave it a name, the name it would always have"

(Eaton, 1995, p. 7). The Creator informed the Man to look carefully at each one, to speak to it its appropriate name. This was the birth of relationship, and the Man who gave the name became the parent, bound to guide and protect. The Lord then goes further to provide Man with additional companionship and fashions woman from the "place of tender emotions in the Man's lowest rib as he sleeps" (p. 7).

The position of animals and birds in this sequence is significant. They are made as companions for the man "that he should not be alone and sad. The Lord brings them to him in the beautiful orchard, one by one, and each is named and recognized as a friend" (Eaton, 1995, p. 7). It is only later that woman is made. The origin of the human pair precedes and follows the making of animals, enveloping the creatures that are to be the humans' companions. They are thus a central part of the story of human origin.

In *The Circle of Creation*, Eaton (1995) wove his way through the proverbs to find that the ancient sages spoke much of animals and plants. There was even commendation of one who "knew the soul of an animal" (Eaton, 1995, p. xi). The Bible features animals significantly in many passages, with many references made to lions and lambs, ravens and reptiles, donkeys, and even dragons. Certain saints are associated with specific animals that appear not only as companions but also as protectors. Peace with animals, especially wild animals, was a sign of God's presence in this world. "And he was with the animals" (Birch & Vischer, 1997, p. 26).

The renaissance and the beginning of the modern era saw the spiritual community with animals and saints all but disappear (Birch & Vischer, 1997). A new awareness of human mastery of the world had emerged, and the world became an object of human knowledge and human will. Fellow creatures began to fade from Christians' field of vision, and the point of view of previous centuries was no longer applicable or even comprehensible. It was dismissed as "the product of a naïve and no longer sustainable way of looking at the world" (1997, p. 27).

Although Christianity may have attempted to erase the pagan gods and their association with animal spirits and animal lore, St. Christopher still bore the head of a dog, and medieval artists continued to rely heavily on animal symbolism to depict the stories and lessons of Christianity (Beck & Katcher, 1996).

As Eaton (1995) introduced the reader to animals that vitally served human need with patience and gentleness, he brought to awareness the importance of animals in the hearts and imagination of the Biblical people. He explained that the stories of Genesis were basic, "which took up great values and presented . . . animals as wonderful creatures of God, beloved by him, and entrusted by him into the care of humanity" (p. 105).

Eaton noted that the scriptures saw that the ideal of animals and people living in harmony had been broken but that a society based on love would again one day be restored (Eaton, 1995, p. 105). "The way to wisdom [is] to look at these animals with love, humility, and a heart open to receive. And here, still more, was a way to find God their Creator" (p. 107). Perhaps animal-assisted therapy is a step toward the reconnecting of this human-animal bond.

Drawbacks of the Biophilia Hypothesis

It is difficult to separate out biophilia, the cultural response to animals of different kinds (Lawrence, 1993), and the effect of social support on both animals and humans (Beck & Katcher, 2003). "The role of both the animal and the 'green' component of the environment cannot be tested apart from multivariate epidemiological studies that would inquire about both an environment and animal impact" (Beck & Katcher, 2003, p. 81).

According to Beck and Katcher (2003), the Biophilia Hypothesis has three limitations. The first is, that the theory does not imply that we have an inborn tendency to maximize the welfare of animals because "our survival for almost all of the past three million years was dependent on sneaking up on animals and killing them" (2003, p. 80). Second, the theory can only be tried in specific cases that prove or disprove the specific instance and cannot be tested in its general form. The third limitation stems from the impossibility of separating out cultural influences from biological ones without extensive testing in diverse social groups. Irvine makes a good point when she says "perhaps we do have a genetic tendency to take an interest in animals, but if that is so, our explanations still need to go further" (2004, p. 32).

RESEARCH INTO THE HUMAN-ANIMAL BOND

Historical Perspectives

Although the term human-animal bond was used prominently in 1979 Scotland, by then the concept had also been articulated by professionals in the United States. Konrad Lorenz, a Nobel Prize-winning ethologist, and Boris Levinson, a psychologist and leading researcher in the concept of animal-assisted psychotherapy, both (articulated this concept) when referring to the link between humans and animals. Internation-al and national conferences in the 1970s and 1980s, along with their published proceedings, brought wide attention to the concept of the human-animal bond, as did media coverage of community animal-assisted activity, therapy programs, and service dog training programs (Hines, 2003).

The need for a research base to support human-animal relationships and how they may be used to facilitate therapy was recognized by a medical doctor, Michael McCulloch. He established the Delta Society in the United States of America in 1977, drawing its membership from many disciplines. It soon became the leading professional organization conducting research on the effects of animals on human health (Bustad, 2001). The mission of the Delta Society is to improve human health through service and therapy animals (Delta Society, 2005).

Dr. McCulloch gave a lecture at an international conference on the human-animal bond that took place at the University of Pennsylvania in October 1981. The following statement is indicative of his strong belief that pets should be recognized as agents of therapy vital to the physical, psychological and social well-being of people: "If pet therapy offers hope for relief of human suffering, it is our professional obligation to explore every available avenue for its use" (as cited in Bustad, 2001, p. 276).

The establishment of the field of human-animal studies was immeasurably influenced through Boris Levinson's two books entitled *Pet-Oriented Child Psychotherapy* (1969) and *Pets and Human Development* (1972). In Forecast for the Year 2000 (1975), he wrote, "Suffering from even greater feelings of alienation than those which are already attacking our emotional health, future man will be compelled to turn to nature and the animal world to recapture some sense of unity with a world that otherwise will seem chaotic and meaningless. . . . Animals will become junior partners and friends, effecting a revolutionary transformation of man's attitudes" (as cited in Hines, 2003, p. 8).

The human-animal bond movement was international in scope from the beginning. It strove to become interdisciplinary, and in the 1970s and early 1980s, centers devoted to the study of human-animal relations were founded. These organizations flourished in at least five countries—United Kingdom, France, Austria, United States of America, and Australia. Others have emerged since those early years. Presentations at national and international interdisciplinary conferences that convened in the 1970s and 1980s gave definition, credibility, and scope to this emerging field (Hines, 2003).

An interdisciplinary approach to the human-animal bond was espoused from its earliest years. However, much of the progress of the field must be attributed to veterinary medicine. "In 1972, The Canadian Veterinary Medical Associations held a successful, landmark meeting on pets in society in Vancouver" (Hines, 2003, p. 9). Other conferences have followed and continue today. However, the concept of the human-animal bond was not really considered mainstream within veterinary medicine until 1999, when it received significant recognition in the *Journal of the American Veterinary Medical Association* (Brown & Silverman, 1999).

Interest of Other Professionals in the Human-Animal Bond

The value of the human-animal bond has slowly become known to other professionals. The concept was introduced to psychiatry, psychology, and sociology by Bossard (1944), Levinson (1962, 1965a & b), Heiman (1967), Corson, Corson, Gwynne, and Arnold (1977), Rynearson (1978), Brickel (1979), and Katcher and Friedmann (1980). From the 1970s until his untimely death in 1985, McCulloch (1981) was a steady voice educating practitioners in human medicine about the value of human-animal interactions, especially those in his specialty of psychiatry.

Schools of social work and public health joined with veterinary schools in organizing early conferences on the human-animal bond. A study by Friedmann, Katcher, Lynch, and Thomas (1980) provided empirical evidence that animal ownership was a factor that contributes to the prevention of disease. This was the first of such studies to be published in a medical journal. In 1991, an entire issue of *Holistic*

Nursing Practice was devoted to and titled, "The Human-Animal Bond: Implications for Professional Nursing." This was done under the editorship of Betty Carmack, a leader in the human-animal bond movement within the nursing profession.

Effects of the Human-Animal Bond in Relation to Human Physical Health

Reports of companion animals positively affecting cardiovascular health also shed validity on the concept of animals as beneficial to human health. Anderson, Reid, and Jennings (1992) reported that pet owners had slightly lower systolic blood pressure, plasma cholesterol, and triglyceride values than non-pet owners had. Patronek and Glickman (1993) reported that pet ownership appears to reduce the incidence of cardiovascular disease because of animals' influence on psychosocial risk factors.

An independent ancillary study to the Coronary Arrhythmia Suppression Trial (CAST), a National Institutes of Health (NIH) clinical trial, found that dog ownership lowered anxiety and is associated with an increased likelihood of one-year survival after a myocardial infarction (Friedmann & Thomas, 1995). Interestingly, the literature suggests that dogs are more valuable for the protection of health than cats are (Friedmann & Thomas, 1995; Serpell, 1991; Siegal, 1990).

Research has shown that the acquisition of a companion animal is associated with lower incidence of minor physical illness as well as an elevated psychological well-being (Serpell, 1991). Companion animals, especially dogs, have also been proven to be beneficial in the maintenance of cardiovascular health. A large-scale study conducted in a cardiovascular risk screening clinic in Australia found that pet owners were at a lower risk for cardiovascular disease (Anderson, Reid & Jennings, 1992). Other studies have also indicated that pet owners have better survival rates and recovery following the incidence of myocardial infarction (Friedmann et al., 1980; Friedmann & Thomas, 1995).

A review of publications of the last ten years reveals an increasing number of articles published in the respected professional journals of a wide variety of disciplines (Hines, 2003). Hooker, Freeman, and Stewart's (2002) historical review on pet therapy research concludes that the use of pets in health institutions has moved from incidental use to research-supported incorporation into programs of care.

SOCIAL AND PSYCHOLOGICAL SUPPORT THEORY

Loneliness–the absence of social support–has always been viewed as a painful and unpleasant sensation. It is no surprise that since time immemorial, societies have used solitary confinement, exile, and social ostracism as methods of punishment. Within the last fifteen years, extensive medical literature has confirmed a strong, positive link between social support and improved human health and survival (Eriksen, 1994; Sherbourne, Meredith, Rogers & Ware, 1992; Vilhajamson, 1993). The precise mechanisms underlying the life-saving effects of social support are still not fully agreed on. However, most agree that the principle benefits arising from supportive social relationships are their ability to buffer, or ameliorate, the deleterious health effects of prolonged or chronic life stress (Ader, Cohen & Felten, 1995).

Effects of the Human-Animal Bond on Human Social Support

Medical researchers and practitioners believe the only relationships that matter are those that exist between closely affiliated human beings. Serpell states, "Despite the growing evidence of recent anthrozoological research, the notion that animal companions might also contribute socially to human health has still received very limited medical recognition" (2000a, p. 16). Yet, findings of numerous studies indicate companion animals are capable of providing people with a form of stress-reducing or stress-buffering support (Allen, Blascovich, Tomaka & Kelsey, 1991; DeMello, 1999; McNicholas & Collis, 1998, 2000; Serpell, 1991; Siegel, 1990).

Companion animals have been found to increase the frequency of human social support in both adults and children (Eddy, Hart & Boltz, 1988; Furman, 1989; Melson, Schwarz & Beck, 1998; Messent, 1983; Rost & Hartmann, 1994). Each of the studies demonstrated that companion animals, especially dogs, act as catalysts for human-human interactions. It is believed this might promote a feeling of social integration.

In one observational study, Messent (1983) discovered that dog owners walking their dogs in parks experienced a significantly higher number of chance conversations with other park users than did those who were walking the same routes without their dogs. Conversations were also found to be longer when their dog was present. This has been called the "ice-breaker" effect, which provides a neutral and safe opening for conversation (McNicholas & Collis, 2000).

Rossbach and Wilson (1992) believed that this ice-breaker effect may be due to a person's likeability increasing because of the presence of a dog. Similar effects have been noted in owners of trained assistance dogs such as guide dogs (Delafield, 1975, as cited in McNicholas & Collis, 2000). Some suggest that assistance dogs may actually be just as valuable in their role as facilitators of social interactions as they are in their role as specialized assistant dogs (Eddy et al., 1988; Hart, Hart & Bergin, 1987; Mader, Hart & Bergin, 1989).

Health advantages associated with pet ownership have tended to center on the nature of the relationship between the owner and pet, and the perception of the pet as a significant relationship and provider of social support and affection. However, McNicholas and Collis (1998) believe there are a number of different mechanisms that could represent various ways in which pets may have a positive impact on well-being and health. In 2000, they conducted a study looking at these suggested mechanisms. They discovered that pets may have a "robust catalysis effect." The pets did enhance social interactions between people, which they connected to increased or strengthened social networks and social provisions. This in turn has the effect of elevating psychological well being.

McNicholas and Collis investigated "the role of pets as social catalysts as a prelude to an investigation of their effects on the size, composition and provision of social networks" (2000, p. 61). They designed a two-part study to further examine Messent's (1983) findings that dogs could act as powerful catalysts of social interaction. They concluded that having a dog present removed or allowed inhibitions to be circumvented when it came to striking up casual conversations (McNicholas & Collis, 2000).

The findings of their study also indicated that the catalysis effect of the dog can have a long-lasting influence on social contact in regard to the robust phenomenon. This was not negated when the dog was absent. "It seems that the presence of a dog on one occasion can act as an 'ice breaker' and provide a focus for subsequent conversations when the dog is absent, in a way that just meeting the same person regularly does not" (McNicholas & Collis, 2000, p. 69). Sarmicanic (2004) noted that companion animals lend authenticity to the performances we put on for others, which could enhance trust in the formation of relationship.

FROM THE HUMAN-ANIMAL BOND TO ANIMAL-ASSISTED THERAPY

The Birth of Animal-Assisted Therapy

For most of human history, animals have occupied a central position in theories concerning ontology and health. Documentary evidence on the historical accounts of people's relationship with animals refer primarily to the lives of the rich and famous (Serpell, 2000a). In *The Pawprints of History*, Coren (2002) wrote about some of history's most prominent figures and their connection with dogs. He tells how Florence Nightingale's chance encounter with a wounded dog led her into the vocation of nursing. He explains how the life of the Fifth Dalai Lama was saved by a dog that shared his bed and how the musician Richard Wagner admitted that one of the arias in his opera *Siegfried* was actually written from inner stirrings evoked by the presence of his dog. Accounts are also told of the dogs that found their way to the battlefield with great military leaders such as Robert the Bruce and Omar Bradley.

Coren (2002) recounts stories of dogs that played a role in inspiring Presidents Lincoln, Roosevelt, Johnson, and Clinton. These animals served not only as loyal pets but also as creative muses. Although there are many more prominent historical figures whose lives were positively affected by animals, the story of Sigmund Freud and his pet chow chows is most pertinent to this literature review. Freud, who developed a fondness for dogs in the last two decades of his life, is considered by many to be the first to incorporate the assistance of dogs in psychotherapy.

Freud redefined human beings by "shifting the explanation of our actions away from simple physiological mechanisms and toward psychological mechanisms" (Coren, 2002, p. 129). The legacy of Freud's relationship with canine companions "resulted in the formation of a new form of psychotherapy (namely animal-assisted therapy) that has very little relationship to the psychoanalytic system that Freud is identified with" (p. 129). His activities with his dogs eventually led to an alternative to psychoanalysis.

Freud often had one of his dogs (usually a chow chow named Jofi) in his office with him while he engaged in psychotherapy sessions. He explained that the dog's response was a good indicator of the patient's state of mind. Freud noted that the presence of the dog seemed to help patients during their session. "This difference was most marked when Freud was dealing with children or adolescents, who seemed more willing to talk openly (especially about painful issues) when the dog was in the room" (Coren, 2002, p. 139). He also noted that the presence of the dog seemed to enhance the comfort level with adults.

Freud recognized that dogs appeared to be unmoved by anything that patients said and came to believe this provided a sense of safety and acceptance. Even when the patient described a very painful or embarrassing moment, the dog did not react, except perhaps with a calm glance in the patient's direction. The dog conveyed a message that anything could be expressed in the therapy room, which in turn provided them with a feeling of reassurance (Coren, 2002). What, in Freud's opinion, the dogs brought to the therapeutic environment closely resembles the qualities inherent in Winnicott's (1965) concept of the holding environment.

The sense of safety provided by the presence of the dog was also noted by Freud, to decrease patient resistance. When his patients were "getting near to uncovering the source of [their] problem. . . . Freud's impression was that this resistance was much less vigorous when the dog was in the room" (Coren, 2002, pp. 139–140). Freud kept meticulous notes on his observations, and his writing eventually encouraged the systematic use of dogs in therapy.

Belief in the socializing and psychotherapeutic properties of animal companionship stretches back to at least the eighteenth century when philanthropic groups in Europe began advocating the introduction of "tame animals" to some of the more progressive mental institutions of the day (Serpell, 2000a). Although during this period of "Enlightenment" having pet animals serve a socializing function for children and the mentally ill was popular, in 1792 the Quakers had already established the York Retreat, an asylum for the "mentally disturbed," in England. It was the first documented case of humans using animals to change the behavior of the mentally ill (Beck & Katcher, 1996; Becker, 2002; Jones, 1985; Ruckert, 1987). By the nineteenth century, the introduction of animals to institutional care facilities was widespread (Serpell, 2000a).

Florence Nightingale was a proponent of animal companionship. In *Notes on Nursing* (1859), she documented the virtues of small pet animals for the sick (as cited in Serpell, 2000a). Bethel, a multibased treatment facility in Bielefield, West Germany, was founded for the treatment of epileptics in 1867. It is now a 5000-patient facility for the treatment of physical and mental disorders. Dogs, cats, horses, birds, farm animals, and even wild animals are still part of the treatment (Beck & Katcher, 1996; Becker, 2002; Bustad, 1981). The first use of animal-assisted therapy in America was at Pawling Army Air Corps Convalescent Hospital in New York from 1944 to 1945. It began when a serviceman requested a dog to keep him company while he recuperated from his war wounds (Beck & Katcher, 1996; Bustad, 1980; Ruckert, 1987).

These early and preliminary experiments in animal-assisted therapy were soon displaced by the rise of scientific medicine during the early part of the twentieth century. Most people date the beginning of the modern interest in human-animal interaction research to the publication of Boris Levinson's (1962) article, "The Dog as Co-Therapist" (Beck & Katcher, 1996; Becker, 2002; Rowan & Thayer, 2000). However, an earlier paper published by James H. S. Bossard (1944) in *Mental Hygiene* also addressed the therapeutic value of dog ownership. Bossard described the roles animals played as "a source of unconditional love; as an outlet for people's desire to express love; as fulfilling a human's desire for exercising power; as a 'teacher' of children on topics such as toilet training, sex education, and responsibility; as social lubricants; and as companions" (Rowan & Thayer, 2000, p. xxvii).

Levinson was the first to formulate animal-assisted therapy into a "self-conscious diagnostic and therapeutic technique" (Beck & Katcher, 1996, p. 133). By extensively publishing his findings in the area of pet-oriented child psychotherapy, Levinson became a leader in developing the presence of animals in the therapeutic setting into an adjunct form of therapy.

Levinson's use of animals as cotherapists followed a startling discovery while working with a young boy who was severely withdrawn and having many problems associated with social contact. On one occasion, Levinson's dog Jingles, not usually permitted in the office when clients were expected, was present because the boy arrived earlier than expected. "The boy began to interact with the dog and to Levinson's surprise spoke to the dog; Levinson had not been able to provoke speech during the previous month. This was the beginning of his research, which has inspired many others to investigate this area" (Edenburg & Baarda, 1995, p. 1).

Jingles seemed to act as an icebreaker with a child Levinson had been unable to reach. The gentle animal softened the child's defenses and provided a focus for communication. With the animal present, Levinson was able to "join in" and establish a rapport. This allowed for the onset of positive therapeutic work (Becker, 2002; Levinson, 1964; Levinson & Mallon, 1997; Ruckert, 1987).

Through documentation, Levinson (1964) demonstrated that pets could be used in the treatment of emotionally disturbed children. He believed a companion animal that displayed unconditional acceptance made the treatment setting a more secure environment for young patients. This, in turn, seemed to assist clients in their ability to express themselves because of what was believed to be an increase in their sense of safety.

Many colleagues met Levinson's work with cynicism and disdain (Beck & Katcher, 1996; Becker, 2002; Serpell, 2000a). Even today, and despite the fact that there is considerable scientific research and supporting data, many professionals continue to question the validity of animal-assisted therapy. Hopefully, with the gradual demise of this medical model mindset, we will return to a more open and holistic view of the potential contribution of animals to human well-being.

Scientists and health-care professionals have put Levinson's theories into practice in scores of therapeutic settings. Corson and Corson (1978) were the first to expand on Levinson's work, implementing the first pet-facilitated therapy program on a psychiatric unit at Ohio State University in 1977. The Corsons selected adolescents who were severely withdrawn for a pilot project aimed at ascertaining the effects of interacting with the canines. Forty-seven of the fifty participants showed marked improvement, with many of those eventually leaving the hospital—the other three had withdrawn from the program near its onset (Beck & Katcher, 1996; Ruckert, 1987).

The animals in Corson and Corson's (1977) study acted as social catalysts, forging a positive link between the patients and the staff. The analyses of patients' interactions with the animals, as well as the human therapists, showed that the patients became less withdrawn, answering therapists' questions sooner and more fully. The patients themselves reported increased self-respect, independence, and confidence (Beck & Katcher, 1996; Becker, 2002).

Pet therapy has proved to be successful with children (Levinson, 1965b), medical patients suffering from depression (McCulloch, 1981), institutionalized mentally ill patients (Corson & Corson, 1980; Siegel, 1962), and elderly people living alone or in nursing homes (Brickel, 1984; Bustad & Hines, 1982; Cusack, 1988; Mugford & McComisky, 1975). Evaluation results from a study on a pet therapy program for cancer patients and those close to them concluded that pets can help individuals in a way people may not be able to (Muschel, 1984). Muschel reported that the animals lessened fears, despair, loneliness, and isolation, thereby increasing their adaptation to a most difficult situation. The positive effects were attributed to the animals' quiet, accepting, and nurturing manner and to the fact that they neither intruded on nor avoided dying patients.

The results of numerous studies have since consistently shown that animals can improve morale, and communication, bolster self-esteem, and increase quality of life. Although there is still considerable skepticism within the scientific community, no one is "laughing" anymore. The evidence is overwhelming, and study after study supports the findings that animals, especially dogs, make us happier, healthier, and more sociable (Allen & Burdon, 1982; Beck & Katcher, 1996; Becker, 2002; Cusack, 1988; Fine, 2000; Knapp, 1998; Muschel, 1985; Ruckert, 1987; Woloy, 1990).

There are many different terms used to describe this adjunct therapy in reading the literature on animal-assisted therapy. Although no standard definition of animal-based interventions exists, the following definitions of animal-assisted therapy and animal-assisted activity have been proposed by the Delta Society, which is the main organization for certifying therapy animals in the United States. These definitions currently appear to be the most widely accepted:

- Animal-Assisted Therapy (AAT): AAT is a goal-directed intervention in which an animal that meets specific criteria is an integral part of the treatment process. AAT is directed and/or delivered by a health/human service professional with specialized expertise, and within the scope of practice of his/her profession. Key features include: specified goal and objectives for each individual; and measured progress.
- Animal-Assisted Activity (AAA): AAA provides opportunities for motivational, educational, recreational, and/or therapeutic benefits to enhance quality of life. AAAs are delivered in a variety of environments by specially trained professionals, paraprofessionals, and/or volunteers, in association with animals that meet spe-

cific criteria. Key features include: absence of specific treatment goal; volunteers and treatment providers are not required to take detailed notes; visit content is spontaneous (Delta Society, n.d. as cited in Kruger, Trachtenberg & Serpell, 2004, p. 4).

Animal-assisted therapy and animal-assisted activities can be grouped together under the more general term, animal-assisted intervention defined here as "any therapeutic intervention that intentionally includes or incorporates animals as part of the therapeutic process of milieu" (Kruger et al., July 2004, p. 4).

The field of animal-assisted interventions currently lacks a unified, widely accepted or empirically supported theoretical framework. A variety of possible mechanisms of action have been proposed or alluded to in the literature that looks at how and why relationships between humans and animals are potentially therapeutic. These focus on the proposed unique intrinsic attributes of animals that appear to contribute to positive changes in clients' self-concepts and behavior and on animals as instruments of cognitive and behavioral change (Kruger & Serpell, 2006).

Animal-Assisted Therapy, Companion Animals, and Trauma

Fox (1981), a veterinarian involved in human-animal bond studies, pointed out that not all people-pet relationships are healthy. Some people may become so involved with their pet that there is a "pathological overattachment and introversion" (p. 38). He questioned whether some people might cease making efforts to go and seek satisfying human relationships because the pet is meeting their needs.

Brown and Katcher (1997, 2001) discovered many people with high pet attachment also have high levels of dissociation. Since dissociation correlates with pet attachment, they believe it is possible that a subset of people highly attached to companion animals would have histories of abuse or trauma. They speculated that traumatized individuals may seek reparative relationships with companion animals as a safe substitute. Their thoughts parallel my own. The trauma I experienced in childhood led me to trust animals more than humans. In reading the work of the previous authors, I questioned whether the attachment bonds built through relationships with companion animals provided a safe way to learn to trust another living being. Could the companion animal form a bridge to a connection with another human?

In pondering Fox's notion that people might not seek human companionship because they have their relational needs met through a pet, I began to question whether this was an actual choice or an instinctive protective behavior. Could people who choose pets over people be doing so in order to reduce their risk of being hurt in relationship? Did those who chose pets over people have past histories of being wounded in human relationships, and were these choices based not so much on preference, but more on the need for safety?

People with high levels of dissociation or trauma tend to be more socially isolated and in more emotional distress (Herman, 1997). Therefore, a dissociative group of people who are highly attached to companion animals may find animal-assisted therapy appealing. I believe it would have been easier for me to enter a therapist's office and develop a working alliance if there had been a welcoming pet to greet me and comfort me. Perhaps it would be easier for others who have been traumatized to take the risk of reaching out for help if they know a furry friend will be there beside them. The growing desire within me to find the answers to these reflections and questions is the foundation of this book.

Chapter 3

UNEARTHING THE TREASURE

The purpose of this book was twofold. The first goal was to discover the role of companion animals in the therapeutic process of counseling and psychology. A phenomenological study was designed, and in-depth semi-structured interviews were conducted with three psychologist-participants who use animals in their therapy settings. The focus of the interviews was their experiences while having a companion animal present during therapy sessions. The second purpose of this book was to apply the themes extracted from the findings of my research to Winnicott's concepts of the holding environment and transitional phenomena (Phillips, 1988).

THE INTERVIEW QUESTIONS

A. The central question guiding this book:

What is the companion animal's role within the therapeutic process of counseling and psychology?

This question was what led to the writing of this book but was not presented to the psychologists/participants during the interviews. I chose to ask two separate interview questions that would not steer or lead participants, thus allowing for the essence of their experience to emerge in its pure form. The interview questions assisted in determining meanings toward the central question but did not taint the responses with the word role.

B. Questions used in the interviews of participants:

1. **What is your experience of having a companion animal present during sessions with clients?**
2. **What value, if any, has been derived from the presence of the companion animal?**

The first question allowed for a personal account of the therapists' experiences of having a companion animal present in therapy sessions with clients. Once the topic had been exhausted, the second question was asked. This question closed the interview and allowed the participants to reflect on whether or not their experiences have indicated that companion animals are, or are not, an asset when present during sessions with clients.

NEED FOR THE PROJECT

The human health benefits derived from relationships with companion animals have attracted a great deal of scientific interest and research. However, there is a need for theoretical conceptualizations in order to understand why the human-pet bond is beneficial. The purpose of this book was to investigate just how companion animals may assist clients within the therapeutic process of counseling and psychology. The central question guiding the research project was aimed at gathering information that would allow me to apply the findings to the contextual framework of object relations theory and Winnicott's (1965) concept of the holding environment and good-enough mother in such a way as to inform the possible role companion animals play within the psychotherapeutic process.

DESCRIPTION OF THE METHODS USED

Qualitative research study is selected when the nature of a research question involves a desire to understand "*what* is occurring," when "the topic needs to be *explored*," when there is a "need to present a *detailed view*," and when a researcher wishes to "study individuals in their *natural setting*" (Creswell, 1998, p. 17).

The operative verb in a phenomenological research study is "describing" (Groenewald, 2004). The word phenomenological is used because this methodology "transforms the world into mere phenomena" (Schmitt, 1967, p. 61). The researcher seeks to understand social and psychological phenomena from the perspectives of the participants involved in the study: "the lived experiences of the people" (Greene, 1997; Holloway, 1997; Kruger, 1988; Kvale, 1996; Maypole & Davies, 2001; Robinson & Reed, 1998) (as cited in Groenewald, 2004, p. 5). This method of qualitative inquiry pursues meanings from experience rather than pure fact (Ashworth, Giorgi & de Koning, 1986).

Phenomenology is concerned with ideas and essences. For the purpose of this study, I chose to use transcendental phenomenological qualitative research methodology. This allowed me to "understand the meaning of experiences of [psychologists] about this phenomenon" (Creswell, 1998, p. 38). In using this method, I was able to study the appearance of things of phenomena just as we see them and as they appear to us in consciousness (Moustakas, 1994). Transcendental moves beyond the everyday to the pure ego where everything is perceived freshly, as if for the first time (Moustakas, 1994).

Farber (1943) lists the functions of transcendental phenomenology (as cited in Moustakas, 1994, p. 49):

1. It is the *first* method of knowledge because it begins with the things themselves, which are the final court of appeal for all we know. It is a logical approach because it seeks to identify presuppositions and "put them out of play."
2. It is not concerned with matters of fact but seeks to determine meanings.
3. It deals with both real essences and possible essences.
4. It offers direct insight into the essence of things, growing out of the self-givenness of objects and reflective description.
5. It seeks to obtain knowledge through a state of pure subjectivity, while retaining the values of thinking and reflecting. (p. 568)

Transcendental phenomenological methodology allowed me to explicate the phenomena in terms of their constituents and possible meanings. From that, I was able to discern the various features of consciousness, which led toward gaining an understanding of the essences of the experience of having a companion animal present during counseling/psychology sessions. These findings were then applied to current theoretical frameworks used in studying the human-animal bond, and to Winnicott's (1953, 1958) object relations-based concepts of transitional relationships and the holding environment.

In order to conduct this phenomenological study, it was "essential that all participants experience[d] the phenomenon being studied" (Creswell, 1998, p. 118). My research participants included three psychologists who use companion animals in their therapy regime. Through their stories, I was able to gain access to the phenomenon found in their lived experience of animal-assisted therapy.

I utilized the suggestion by Kirby and McKenna (1989) and considered research participants to be collaborators and researchers themselves. They each held equal status with me, the prime researcher. Prior to my initial contact, I reviewed an interview checklist to remind me of all I needed to include in our conversation (*see* Appendix B). This helped me to fix my attention on what I wanted to include in our discussion prior to dialoguing with potential participants. It also ensured all participants knew "enough about the research focus to want to participate, were able to share in the information gathering process and ultimately, to see themselves in the final report of the study" (Kirby & McKenna, 1989, p. 104).

Creswell (1998) suggested that the initial step in a phenomenological research project is the self-reflection of the researcher. Thus, I began the first chapter of this book by integrating current literature on the effects of companion animals on psychological and spiritual health with my lived experience of having a dog as companion during my difficult childhood years. This in turn explained my current interest and musings in the area of animal-assisted therapy.

ETHICAL CONSIDERATIONS

Confidentiality

All participants interviewed signed an agreement to be interviewed that included a confidentiality clause and assurance of anonymity. These were kept securely throughout the process. Confidentiality of participants and names given in the interview were maintained through the use of pseudonyms. The names of companion animals were also kept confidential through the use of pseudonyms. Participants were supplied with copies of the transcription and were asked to inform me of any corrections. They were also given the right to ask that parts of the interview be excluded. The interview tapes and transcriptions were kept secure at all times in a locked cabinet. The computer used to store written transcriptions required a password. The person hired to transcribe the tapes signed an agreement of confidentiality and had no previous knowledge of the research or participants (*see* Appendix D). The "independent judge" (Hycner, 1985, p. 289) was an individual not involved in the study who was used as "competent other." This person's role was to competently interpret, describe, and evaluate the findings in order to ensure validity (Eisner, 1991, p. 112). The judge was an outsider to the study and signed a form in regard to confidentiality (*see* Appendix G).

The participants were informed they had the right to rescind their agreement and withdraw from this project at any time. The audiotapes from the interviews were destroyed following completion of the study. Transcripts will be kept securely for five years in order to allow for possible journal submissions of research. Participants will be informed if submissions do occur.

Ethical Responsibility

Ethics approval to carry out the study contained within this book was obtained through the St. Stephen's College Ethics Review Committee. Written confirmation of this was dated June 1, 2006. The interviews began in June 2006 and were completed July 2006.

COLLECTION OF INFORMATION

Participants

As stated in Chapter 1, participants were selected on the basis of having had experiences with and without a companion animal present while conducting therapy sessions with clients. Suitable candidates were found through referral from the project manager of The Chimo Project based in Edmonton, Alberta. This research-based program works toward identifying ways that animals can effectively be used in the treatment of mental illness, while also promoting the study of animal-assisted therapy. The Chimo Project's manager and director are currently researching ways to incorporate animal-assisted therapy into the curriculum of schools of psychiatry, psychology and other training for professionals and hospitals.

The Chimo Project was the first in Canada to implement a program that brings psychotherapists and their clients together with selected and screened animals in order to document and prove that animal-assisted therapy is beneficial for persons with mental illness and/or psychological dysfunction (Urichuk & Anderson, 2003). All therapists involved in the project must attend a course on animal-assisted psychotherapy offered through The Chimo Project.

Counselors, psychologists, and psychiatrists involved in this project can use their own companion animal if it is able to pass a temperament test, as well as a specific behavior test designed by The Chimo Project. The animal also has to be cleared as healthy and suitable through veterinarian screening. Therapists wanting to be involved in The Chimo Project, but who do not have suitable animals of their own, can utilize a volunteer base of handlers and their dogs; they hope to add teams of handlers with cats in the near future. The volunteers are put through a training program, and their animals must meet the criteria to work as therapy pets. The team of handler and dog is then assigned to a therapist. They become part of the treatment plan, and the handler brings the therapy animal to regular sessions with clients. The handler remains with his or her pet at all times to ensure the animal's needs are met.

Selection of Participants

Purposive sampling, which is a nonprobability form of sampling, was used to identify the primary participants (Welman & Kruger, 1999). This form of sampling allows researchers to choose the primary participants based on their judgment and the purpose of the enquiry. Patton (2002) described this form of sampling in the following statement: "The logic and power of purposeful sampling lie in selecting information-rich cases for study in-depth. . . . Information-rich cases are those from which one can learn a great deal about issues of central importance to the purpose of the inquiry. . . . Studying information-rich cases yields insights and in-depth understanding rather than empirical generalization" (Patton, 2002, p. 230).

Three "expert participants" were found, which means they had a companion animal present during their therapy sessions with clients

(Morse & Richards, 2002, p. 34). Prior to the interviews, each participant was made aware of the purpose of the study and was assured the findings would not involve the content of any of their therapy sessions—only their experience of having a dog present. It was explained that this study would be based on what role the companion animals may have in the therapeutic process; the information on the interactions with the animals was the focus, not confidential client information.

In order to ensure ethical research, I used an informed consent. This document included the following specifics as suggested by Groenewald (2004):

- Participants were informed that they would be participating in a research study.
- The purpose of the research was explained, as well as the procedures.
- An explanation of the voluntary nature of research participation was given.

In discussions surrounding companion animals, emotions are often stirred as memories arise (Nicoll, 2005). Some emotions can be uncomfortable; participants were informed of this possibility. All three psychologists stated that they knew how conversations involving pets can bring up memories; however, they felt there would be little risk to them personally because they would be reflecting on their experience as a therapist working with a pet in the room during sessions. They would not be delving into past or present personal issues. They were, however, told support would be available if needed from the coordinators of the Master of Arts in Pastoral Psychology and Counseling (MAPPC) program, both of whom are counselors. All participants stated they had supervisors or coworkers who could assist them if difficult emotional issues arose.

The benefits of participating in this project were discussed and included: being able to play a role in furthering research toward animal-assisted therapy; aiding in seeking out new understanding into how animal-assisted therapy could be applied as an adjunct therapy by psychologists and counselors; and exploring the role the companion animals have played in their practice by having the opportunity to reflect and share their stories.

The procedures used to protect the participants' confidentiality and anonymity were discussed, and they were made aware of the fact that they had the right to stop the research at any time. Because this study was conducted at the time I was completing my thesis project, participants were informed that they would be able to contact the coordinators of the MAPPC program at St. Stephen's College if they had any concerns.

The Interviews

All three interviews took place in the participants' offices, where they routinely see clients. All three of the participants were registered psychologists. Two of the therapists used dogs (Cloey, Digger, and Bobby), and one used a cat (Lucky). Along with having experience using her pet in the therapy room, one of the participants also had experience visiting clients and patients as a volunteer in two pet-therapy programs while attending university. These programs ran in a cancer center and a woman's shelter in eastern Canada. She stated that during those times her pet Labrador retriever (Harry) brought a great deal of joy and comfort to both adults and children. The first two psychologists work within an organization involved in The Chimo Project. The third participant is in private practice and sees all age groups for individual, marital, and family therapy.

The two participants who are involved in The Chimo Project received training in animal-assisted activities that they incorporated into a cognitive behavioral treatment plan. Their clientele consists of at-risk adolescents between the ages of twelve and sixteen. Some clients are seen as outpatients; the more severe cases are in residential programs.

The first participant, whom I will call Therapist A, follows a cognitive behavioral theoretical framework. In 1993, she became involved in a pet-therapy program with her mother. They brought their Labrador retrievers to visit children at a woman's shelter. In subsequent years, they took their dogs to visit at a cancer center in the city where they resided. She remembers one of the cancer patients saying, "When I came here I thought it was going to be this very cold-hearted place and then I saw you and your dog here." The participant added, "It makes me teary because I'm amazed . . . people are drawn to the dogs, especially if they're worried or highly anxious."

Once she began working as a clinical therapist at an adolescent treatment center, she set up a pet-visitation program. Although this program was not as structured as The Chimo Project, they would "integrate cognitive behavioral therapy and motivational aspects of therapy to bring kids around and do some rapport building." Upon completing her doctoral studies and moving to another city, she was "thrilled" to find out that her new employer was involved with animal-assisted therapy through The Chimo Project, "and they were quite game and enthusiastic [for her] to bring [her cat, Lucky] in."

Therapist A's office was in the lower level of the facility. It was windowless and quite small. She had a desk with a computer on the left wall, a table with a bowl of candy on the right wall, and a couch for clients at the back against the wall. On the left side of the couch, in the corner, a small wall unit held her cat's toys and brushes. These were kept in reach for the children to use during appointments when they did activities with the cat. She stated that she keeps her office dimly lit in order to "enhance the relaxed atmosphere for both my clients and the cat."

I was able to observe a therapy session between Therapist A and a twelve-year-old boy while her cat was present. Permission was granted within the agency where she worked and through The Chimo Project. Although my observations are not included as part of this research, the experience allowed me to witness animal-assisted therapy first hand.

Upon entering the room, the young boy immediately began to look for the cat as he went to the couch at the back of the room and sat down. As soon as the cat was let out of his kennel, Therapist A put on his harness. Lucky then headed straight to the boy and hopped up on his lap. The boy immediately began stroking the cat and commented on the cat's purring. For the boy, this purring seemed to act as a validation of how much the cat liked him.

I was taken by the cat's ability to soothe the child. At one point in the session, the cat moved off the boy to stretch. The boy soon started fidgeting and began to act agitated. However, it was not long before the cat returned and lay down beside the boy. Once the boy began stroking the cat, he again became calm.

While observing the therapy session, I was aware of a sense of peacefulness that seemed to evolve from the presence of the animal. I was also extremely moved by the animal-child interaction that took place. There was a bond of mutual caring, and the affection was evident throughout the session.

The second interview was in the office of Therapist B, who is also a psychologist. When asked what theoretical framework he followed, he wrote, "My framework was a combination of CBT [cognitive behavioral therapy] and Client Centered. In AAT [animal-assisted therapy], it was apparent that '[Digger]' or '[Cloey]' were utilized as the 'Carl Rogers' providing that environment of unconditional positive regard, while in that context, I would incorporate some CBT techniques during our session."

This participant has never owned a companion animal and uses volunteer teams of handlers and their dogs. He stated, "I love dogs. The only problem with me is I'm very allergic to dogs. . . . I have . . . to take extra precaution. I always wish I had a dog, but my allergies would not allow me to have that."

When asked how he liked working with volunteer handlers and their dogs, he said, "they know their pet very well. I don't have to worry about that. I'm just kind of the facilitator." Later he added, "You have to give the handlers a lot of credit, being strong, to sometimes hear about some of the things, and show that empathy themselves. To kind of be in the moment and to just help me out – help me to help them [the clients] express themselves."

Therapist B had a large office with a window in the right wall, up near the ceiling. There were shelves on the bottom of this wall, with various articles used in his practice. His desk, which held a computer, and chair were situated on the left wall. There was a movable chair available for clients or the dog handler, a large couch against the front wall, and a big bean bag cushion on the floor for the kids to use if they chose to. There was no animal present during our interview. I was taken with the fact that this man had never owned a pet, yet had such a passion for animal-assisted therapy. He told me his interest began when he observed a therapy session where there was an animal present. He stated:

> A former colleague/mentor of mine actually allowed me to sit in on a session where there was an animal present. I immediately noticed a very different kind of feeling from the therapy perspective. My feeling was that the guardedness on my part, and also the client, the feeling of tension in the air was pretty much eliminated – diminished. I instantly felt a lot more comfortable myself just being in the role of an observer and note taking; I felt a lot more relaxation. Just playing with the dog when the dog approached me alleviated a whole lot of feeling/tension. . . . Just normal feelings of stress were alleviated. I thought to myself, "That's a very interesting tool to really help with issues regarding resistance in therapy."

Prior to his experience working in animal-assisted therapy, Therapist B was unaware of the powerful impact it would have on clients. He added, "Although I can't put statistics on what I see, can I say it makes a positive change? Yes!"

The third interview was held in the office of Therapist C, whose clientele consisted of children, teens, and adults. This registered psychologist is primarily a narrative therapist but says, "I've been around for so long that I've done so many things . . . a lot of my stuff is interpersonal systems theory and narrative theory." He and his golden retriever have worked together for seven and one half years. He does not use cognitive behavioral therapy techniques in his practice and does not follow any animal-assisted activity treatment guidelines. He believes the dog's presence adds to the therapeutic encounter. When asked what the dog provides, he stated, "I really think in terms of the general quality of the environment and one's sense of safety in the environment and comfort is probably the contribution."

Bobby, the therapy dog, greeted me at the door when I arrived at the office, and was present throughout the interview. Therapist C's office was quite large, with windows along the back wall. His desk was on the far left and was separated from the area where he saw clients by a large comfortable couch. He also had chairs situated around the couch and coffee tables, much like the sitting area of a home. Along with individual therapy, this psychologist does marriage and family therapy, and requires more space. Even though the office was quite large the presence of the dog brought a "homey" feel to the setting.

Therapist C has his dog present during all sessions unless clients request otherwise or the dog's behavior indicates he would like to leave (i.e. the dog goes to the door and signals he wants it opened). His dog roams freely around the entire office and will at times attend sessions with other therapists and their clients. Therapist C got involved in animal-assisted therapy because "I was working a lot with children and I felt the dog would be an asset working with children." Therapist C also practices equine-assisted therapy. He explained that the horses are quite different from what he does with his dog in office. He states, "the horses in the program are used as feedback for people . . . we have activities specifically developed for the horses and the people to do together, and the responses of the horses give feedback to the people in terms of emotional dynamics and relationships."

Therapists A and B only use animal-assisted therapy with a selected number of clients. Therapist A stated she had a three-month waiting list for clients requesting animal-assisted therapy but is cognizant of not overtaxing her cat. Therapist B relies on volunteers, so his ability to provide animal-assisted therapy depends on the availability of handlers and their animals.

Two of the interviewees had animals present and one did not. The interviews with the pets present seemed to be more relaxed and comfortable. I wondered if the animals were "grounding" everyone in the room, giving the sense all was okay. I considered whether if this feeling of comfort was perhaps due to my own love for animals or the therapeutic presence of the individual therapists. Was it the presence of the animals that affected the environment, or was it a combination of all three variables? I was excited to gather and review the data to determine what themes would emerge.

Methods Used In Collection of Information

Interviews

Participants signed two consent forms prior to the onset of our conversation. The first form was the consent to be interviewed and included information on confidentiality (*see* Appendix C). The second form was the consent to be audiotaped (*see* Appendix D). One semistructured in-depth interview per participant was conducted and audiotaped. Each interview lasted one and one half to two hours in length. The interviews were continued until the topic was exhausted or saturated and [comprised questions] directed to the participant's experiences, observations, feelings, beliefs, and convictions (Morse & Field, 1995, p. 94). The specific phenomena focused on were the psychologists' experiences of having a companion animal present during therapy sessions.

In order to allow the stories to emerge, participants were asked the interview questions, rather than the central research question. This prevented participants from focusing on the role of companion animals and allowed the experience itself to emerge. Rich descriptions of phenomena and their settings were used as a "ground stone" from which to discover the underlying commonalities that mark the essential core of the phenomenon (Groenewald, 2004; Seamon, 2000).

Central Research Question:

What is the companion animal's role within the therapeutic process of counseling and psychology?

Interview Questions:

1. What is your experience of having a companion animal present during sessions with clients?

2. What value, if any, has been derived from the presence of the companion animal?

Two forms of bracketing were used during the interviews. Bracketing is a deliberate and purposeful opening to the phenomenon by suspending or "bracketing out" the researcher's own presuppositions (Moustakas, 1994). In the first form, I focused on what went on within the participants and asked them to describe the lived experiences free from intellectual constructs. Then I asked the participants to set aside their experiences about animal-assisted therapy and share reflection on its value. The second form of bracketing involved the bracketing of my own preconceptions, which allowed me to enter into the individual's "life-world" (Moustakas, 1994, p. 48). I utilized my "self" as an experiencing interpreter to understand the world from the participants' point of view (Groenewald, 2004).

Audiorecorded interviews were stored on separate cassettes with an assigned interview code. The person hired to transcribe the tapes signed a consent form agreeing to keep the content of the tapes, and the tapes themselves, safe and secure while in his or her possession. The transcriber had no previous or current knowledge of the identity of the participants and agreed to confidentiality in regard to the content of the interview tapes (*see* Appendix F).

Participants were asked to fill out a "Perspectives and Demographics" form at the end of the interview (*see* Appendix E). This provided additional information on the participants in the event it was felt to be pertinent to the study. The questionnaire was left with the participants to fill out at their leisure, along with a self-addressed stamped envelope.

Methods for Storing Information

AUDIORECORDINGS OF INTERVIEWS. Each interview was on a separate tape, labeled with an assigned code, and kept in a locked cabinet separate from the participants' names so that the tapes would remain anonymous as well as confidential. The tapes were listened to immediately after the interview and, once transcribed, were again listened to in order to correct any omissions or errors. They were then sent off to the participants for review. No corrections were needed, but one participant clarified the names of authors about whom she had spoken. The participants' names did not appear on any of the stored transcripts. Interview transcriptions were stored electronically on two hard drives, on disc, and on hard copy and were only accessible through computer password or locked cabinet.

RESOURCE MATERIAL. I opened files with divisions for the various interviews and stored them on hard copy in a locked file cabinet. These included the informed consent agreement, notes made during the interview, additional information that the participant offered during the interview, completed "Perspectives and Demographics" forms; notes made during the data analysis process (e.g. units of meaning into themes), the draft transcription and analysis of the interview that was presented to the participants for validation, the confirmation of correctness and/or commentary by the participant about the transcript and analyses of the interview, subsequent communication between the participants and myself, and notes from an independent judge who volunteered to verify the units of relevant meanings (Groenewald, 2004; Hycner, 1985).

Information storage included the use of a computer hard drive, disc, written card file, and a hard copy filing system to organize and document findings during the literature search. Information found on the internet was documented in my computer and on a disc. Computer access required a password, and a locked file cabinet was used to hold hard copies of confidential material.

ANALYSIS AND INTERPRETATION OF INTERVIEWS

"The phenomenological method's objective is to describe the full structure of an experience lived, or what that experience meant to those who lived it" (Sadala & Adorno, 2002, p. 289). An analysis of the structure of a phenomenon within a context is one of the outcomes of phenomenological research. The process I used to analyze the information was guided by phenomenology's fundamental ideas and included the following steps.

1. Bracketing and Phenomenological Reduction

This is a deliberate and purposeful opening by the researcher to the phenomenon by suspending or "bracketing out" the researcher's own presuppositions. Previous meanings and interpretations or theoretical concepts were held in check in order to enter the unique world of the participant (Creswell, 1998; Moustakas, 1994).

2. Delineating Units of Meaning Relevant to the Research Question

This step involved explicating those statements that are seen to illuminate the researched phenomenon. These were extracted while consciously bracketing out presuppositions in order to avoid inappropriate subjective judgments (Creswell, 1998; Groenewald, 2004; Hycner, 1985). This process of the data analysis was done by placing the transcribed interviews in column one of a two-column format in a computer document. Column two was used to hold "units of meaning relevant to the research question." Each of the transcribed interview's "units of meaning" was highlighted in a different shade and held the page number it was found on. The exact words from the transcription were used (*see* Appendix H). An independent judge verified the units of relevant meaning as a reliability check. After this, Hycner's (1985) suggestion was followed in order to eliminate redundancies: the list of units of relevant meaning were reviewed, and those that were clearly redundant to others previously listed were eliminated.

3. Clustering of Units of Meaning to Form Themes

While again bracketing presuppositions, the lists of units of meaning were examined to elicit the essence of meaning units within the holistic context (Hycner, 1985; Moustakas, 1994). Clusters of themes were formed by "grouping units of meaning together" (Groenewald, 2004, p. 19). Significant topics were then identified which could also be called units of significance. This was again done on a two-columned computer document. The first column held the extracted units of meaning; the second column was used to further flesh out the essence in order to group together units of meaning.

These units of meaning were then grouped together on a third document in which clusters of units of meaning were further narrowed down. The units of meaning remained in different shades, with the page number of the transcription attached, in order to ease the process when extracting thick descriptions for validation. Initially, there were sixty-one units of meaning. The number of times a meaning was noted was calculated in order to understand how often particular meanings had arisen—been discussed or referred to (*see* Appendix I). The clusters were further grouped together and seventeen themes emerged. These were further grouped into five themes (*see* Appendix J).

4. Summarize Each Interview, Validate and Modify

This was done through summarizing and incorporating all the themes elicited from the data in order to give a holistic context. This involved the reconstruction of the inner world of experience of the subject. Each individual had his or her own way of experiencing temporality, spatiality, and materiality, but each of these coordinates needed to be understood in relation to the others and to the total "inner world" (Groenewald, 2004; Hycner, 1985). This involved putting myself in the shoes of the other in order to become familiar with the lenses they may have used to gain perception of their lived experience.

This step of the process involved the formation of more concise themes. It was a rather lengthy process as I worked to further flesh out the essence that arose from the experiences of the participants while also working toward the avoidance of redundancy in themes. The number of themes was further culled into four (*see* Appendix K). These four themes described the essence of the participants' experiences of having a companion animal present during sessions with clients. A validity check was done by the independent judge, who was not involved in the research project. The judge agreed with the findings and no modifications were needed.

5. Return to the Participant with the Summary and Themes

Hycner suggests that "an excellent experiential 'validity check' is to return to the research participant with the written summary and

54 *The Role of Companion Animals in Counseling and Psychology*

themes and engage in a dialogue with this person concerning what the researcher has found so far" (1985, p. 291). In doing so, the research participants were able to agree or disagree that the essence of their interviews had been accurately and fully captured. Findings were also presented at an Animal-Assisted Therapy Interest Group meeting. All feedback concurred with the themes as extracted.

6. Modifying Themes and Summary

With the new input gained from the research participants' review of the summary and themes, procedures from step one to four were repeated. Upon completion, all of the information was reviewed as a whole, and modifications to themes were made as necessary.

7. Extracting General and Unique Themes from All the Interviews and Observations Followed by a Composite Summary

This step involved looking for the themes that were common to most or all of the interviews. "This procedure requires the phenomenological viewpoint of eliciting essences as well as the acknowledgement of existential individual differences" (Hycner, 1985, p. 292).

Through the use of shading on the various transcriptions (*see* Appendix I), I was able to find the themes common to all of the interviews, while also noticing unique qualities among the themes. For example, each of the participants saw animal-assisted therapy as an adjunct therapy. However, two integrated the companion animals into their practice of cognitive behavioral therapy; the third felt the presence of the animal was the adjunct therapy.

8. Contextualization of Themes

The final step involved writing a composite summary that reflected the context from which the themes emerged (Groenewald, 2004; Hycner, 1985; Moustakas, 1994).

9. Composite Summary

The composite summary "describe[d] the 'world' in general, as experienced by the participants" (Hycner, 1985, p. 294). At the end of each summary, I noted any significant individual differences.

TRUSTWORTHINESS OF RESULTS

Eisner's (1991) standards for establishing the credibility of the study were used: structural corroboration, consensual validation, and referential adequacy (as cited in Creswell, 1998). Structural corroboration involved relating multiple types of data to support or contradict the interpretation. I looked for "recurring behaviors or actions and consider[ed] disconfirming evidence and contrary interpretations" (p. 198).

Consensual validation seeks the opinion of others who can competently interpret, describe, and evaluate the data. An individual not directly involved in the research acted as a "competent other" (Eisner, 1991, p. 112) or "independent judge" (Hycner, 1985, p. 289). In doing so, this person supplied referential adequacy, which "suggests the importance of criticism" (Creswell, 1998, p. 198). The goal of criticism is described as "illuminating the subject matter and bringing about more complex and sensitive human perceptions and understanding" (p. 198). The independent judge signed a confidentiality agreement (*see* Appendix G). The judge was then supplied with the transcriptions and findings, which were shredded upon completion of the task.

Steps taken were relistening to tapes along with the transcription and using the bracketing method while doing so, participants' receiving a copy of the text in order to validate that their perspectives regarding the phenomena studied were accurate, and verifying the clusters of units of meanings and the themes through an independent judge. Exploring procedures included clarifying researcher bias through a "competent other" or independent judge, writing detailed and thick descriptions, and having participants review the summary and themes (Creswell, 1998; Hycner, 1985).

As collaborators in the research, participants were free to comment on both the presentation of the information and the analysis and suggest changes if necessary. They were invited to make suggestions for changes regarding their own personal "experiences" to ensure that it accurately reflected what they had shared through their narrative.

Chapter 4

ANALYZING THE FIND

Four major themes arose from the information collected through interviews with participants who use animal-assisted therapy in their practices of counseling and psychology. Each theme will be explained in this chapter, along with the subthemes held within.

The first theme of ***enhanced therapeutic alliance/relationship*** suggested the animals increased client trust and acted as a catalyst for healing. The second theme involved the animals' creating an ***enhanced therapeutic environment***. Encapsulated within this theme were the notions that companion animals provide a warm, friendly, safe environment; extend unconditional acceptance; foster nurturing; and enhance creativity in both the therapist and the client.

Contained within the third theme of ***enhanced professional practice*** was evidence of how participants used the animals to complement their practices of cognitive behavioral therapy, person-centered therapy, narrative therapy, interpersonal therapy, and marriage and family systems therapy. The animals also appeared to enhance the participants' sense of well-being while working. The fourth theme extracted was based on evidence indicating that the animals in therapy helped in ***creating a sense of sacredness***.

THEME I: ENHANCED THERAPEUTIC ALLIANCE/RELATIONSHIP

Enhancing Trust

Having a companion animal present in the room acted to increase

Analyzing the Find   57

the level of trust clients felt toward their psychologist. When one participant was asked whether an animal would make her seem less threatening with children, she responded by saying,

> *"Oh yes! I'm sure I appear somewhat fun, and I probably appear like a softer person because kids, the majority of kids who come here, have already had the experience in the system with therapy. And especially when I tell them that my background is psychology. I'm sure some of them go "Oh, my God!!" So I think they think that I'm probably more relaxed, or I'm a softer person. Not softer in terms of like boundaries and that kind of thing. . . . So I believe that they probably respond differently."*

This trust has an icebreaker effect during initial sessions and served as a bridge, allowing for what was referred to as "rapport building." Participants looked forward to their appointments, and attendance was never an issue. They found clients to be more engaged and experienced less resistance during sessions. During the interviews, participants mentioned that the animal facilitated the relationship closeness thirty-two times, and the client's positive attitude towards therapy was mentioned twenty-eight times.

In the following excerpts, participants discussed the icebreaker effect of the companion animal during initial sessions.

> *"I think that it is far easier for kids to interact with [Lucky] initially than it is for them to interact with me, because pets of course are full of that unconditional positive regard. They love you even if you're having a bad day, and they don't care if your hair is messy and they don't care if you're weeping on the couch. . . . But I think it's far easier for them to be looking at [Lucky] and talk to you than it may be with me initially. I think that's definitely beneficial."*

* * * * *

> *"We're going to talk about things that are painful, that are uncomfortable—they're very reluctant to talk about. In a lot of ways it [animal-assisted therapy] facilitates a sense of trust. . . . There are just aspects in animal-assisted therapy that will provide a very valuable catalyst in strengthening things like a rapport and trust."*

The client's increased attendance and compliancy were spoken of thirty-eight times during the interviews. One therapist working with adolescents stated, "*Of course kids were more likely to come to their appointments when the cat was there.*" Other similar comments were made:

"When their time comes for their appointments, they're usually like 'yes.' They come out and they run downstairs." One spoke of the data showing that her clients state they attend sessions more because of the animal:

> *"Well I know for a fact that it brings them to therapy. They're more likely to come and see me. They've actually written that when they've done The Chimo Project survey – we do one after every session."*

Another psychologist involved in the treatment of troubled adolescents had this to say about his experience of *"less resistance from clients:"*

> *"Noticing a real difference in the way a client approaches therapy; [it] is a lot different, from "Oh, I have to see [therapist] in session" to "Wow. I can't wait to see [therapist] and [Digger] in session." That is a really significant difference."*

In regard to the companion animal acting as a "bridge" while also decreasing resistance to therapy, the following statement was made:

> *". . . I had a child since last year; she would be very sporadic in session. . . . Basically she would range from being very involved and engaged in session to being very defensive. This being defensive presented with things like silliness, not listening to my dialogue, disengagement, or outright refusal to sit. With the addition of [Cloey] the client was always looking forward to a session. It wasn't so much that she would use [Cloey], because she is very capable at using [Cloey] as a distracter for me too. . . . But she actually was very engaged in the session; was very 'on' – had very positive feelings. And I noticed another thing with successive sessions – I would notice the warmth would generalize towards me."*

When a companion animal is present during therapy, the psychologists noticed that their client's level of engagement increased. As one participant explained,

> *"You'll notice differences in affect. You'll notice differences in the emotive verbal and nonverbal behavior where a client may present in normal circumstances as emotionally flat, very reserved – withdrawn. With the addition of say [Digger] or [Cloey], you see them animated; you see engaging."*

The most powerful effect of the enhanced level of trust was the enhanced disclosure and a deepening of the therapeutic work. This was mentioned a total of fifty-nine times. The participants spoke of clients being able to finally openup to their pain. The animals allowed for the sense of safety needed for vulnerable hurting individuals to risk disclosure. As one participant stated, "*I do envy the two dogs. I envy [Cloey] and [Digger] because they have that capacity to just help people, to bring down those barriers.*"

Catalyst for Enhanced Healing

The companion animal acting as a catalyst for enhanced healing was mentioned seventy-seven times during the interviews. The word catalyst is used in this study to mean an encounter that held the essence of transformation. The animal seemed to supply the chemistry needed to touch off a sort of alchemistic process in the client's growth.

> "*This one client . . . this girl would not talk, share. She would just clam up prior to this . . . imagine a girl like fighting to maintain something inside her; keep something in . . . her reaction was that she was being violated. Then this dog came in. . . . That was my first sign of life. Wow. This is great. This is amazing. This is what makes therapy a very powerful tool . . . it's difficult to have an impact on these kids. . . . But [Digger] . . . does wonderful work that just helps the soul to feelings regarding disclosure, emotional issues.*"

One of the participants would allow clients to bring their own dogs into sessions if he felt it would be beneficial. He told the story of a young girl who used her own dog as a catalyst for healing. This gentle creature provided the comfort and safety needed for the psychologist to help this severely wounded young girl.

> *A teenager came, and she had a big black German shepherd. . . . And she [the young girl] had really been mistreated by humans, and she brought this dog . . . she's here [sitting–he points to the couch], and this big German shepherd sat right on her lap, and the questions that I asked she would look out around behind the German shepherd and answer the questions. And what a sense of how unsafe she felt and how much that dog was needed by her.*"

Clients tell stories related to the animals in their past. Often these stories reveal a history of their own abuse or the abuse of an animal.

> *I guess that's one thing that any clinician who's offering therapy will expect – I'm talking about animal-assisted therapy – there are stories that*

will come up out of the past. I find that hard to deal with as well. So I do my best to help them process it, and if I need to consult with the supervisor then I'll do that as well.

A friendly animal can bring comfort to those who have experienced trauma. In a womean's shelter, a dog's presence can often allow people tactile opportunities to feel warmth and safety.

"It was [in] a women's shelter that there would be children that would come into our program . . . who were, acute[ly] traumatized or who had just been taken from their family home the night before or fled with their mother to the shelter. . . . I thought it would be beneficial to bring [Harry] into the house. . . . I will never forget the day that I brought him in for the first time and literally eight children went around him in a circle and began to like pet him and talk to him and kiss him and hug him. It was amazing just to see that."

The animals seemed to bring the sense of safety needed to confront difficult memories. In the following excerpt, a participant discusses how a friendly therapy dog helped him to reach a severely wounded young boy.

"Another young boy . . . had issues regarding family discord – removal from the family – detachment and abandonment. He had a lot of issues regarding trust. He did not trust the people around him. He did not trust me. I would do whatever I could to try and facilitate some sort of a dialogue that was genuine, but a lot of the answers – the responses – that came from this boy were very shallow and very – as a matter of fact, how should I say this, lack of any substance, genuineness. . . . Emotionally flat is also another aspect. Because of this, there was a stagnation in our therapeutic progress. I interjected the idea of having animal therapy because he mentioned that he'd had a dog. . . . And sure enough. . . . I was really happy to see him jump right into [Digger] and just pet him. I think animal-assisted therapy has really – that has been our – for me and this one boy – has been a smoking gun in therapy. It's been really, really working."

All of the participants spoke of victims of trauma who had received comfort from their animals. They had not "shut-down," like many victims do, and it was thought the animals played a role in assisting them to remain connected.

Analyzing the Find 61

*"So if anyone's feeling helpless, it would have been those two gals for sure.
. . . They were great candidates for animal-assisted therapy because they
had pets in the past. They had empathy. Their mom, she was encouraging
their [relationship] with pets. . . . But they weren't shut down either,
which is the amazing thing. They were another two of the kids that were
all over [Harry]."*

Children and adolescents grieving the loss of their pets due to placement outside of the family home benefited from animal-assisted therapy. One psychologist stated that having an animal allows them to begin to open up. *"It leads to all kinds of questions about what's happened in this child's past."* One participant stated,

"I had a client at the beginning of this week whose social worker actually requested that she participate in animal-assisted therapy. She's a young woman and she's left her pets behind with her grandmother and she loves to come and see [Lucky] because she's missing her pets."

The companion animals decreased sadness and improved the clients' sense of hope. As one psychologist said, *"I think that their [clients] general sense of well-being is enhanced. And so therefore, they're in an ego state or a mental, emotional state that they can more easily do work."* One participant commented on his experience of the dog's helping a young girl build her confidence.

"The client was very withdrawn initially; socially withdrawn. Didn't want to share . . . didn't have a lot of confidence. And I . . . bring [Digger] out into the classroom setting to give a little lesson to the school . . . in a very safe, gentle way, about how [Digger] is helping kids, helping others. . . . And she even got to do demonstrations performing certain tricks for the classroom, with [Digger]. . . . The client was very happy, very swelled up. We would build up confidence."

THEME II: ENHANCED THERAPEUTIC ENVIRONMENT

Warm, Friendly, Safe Environment

A companion animal's presence during sessions brought a sense of warmth and safety. This was mentioned ninety-four times, so it was obviously an important observation made by the participants. From the interviews, it was very apparent that a companion animal often

62   *The Role of Companion Animals in Counseling and Psychology*

supplies the needed ingredients to make the therapeutic encounter occur in a less-threatening atmosphere. The following excerpts are examples:

> *"The first thing that I will say is the degree of comfort that the animal creates for the client. Coming to see the psychologist is somewhat of an anxious process. You know you're going to be talking about something that is creating intense feelings for you most likely – something that is not going well in your life. A lot of people are very anxious in coming and to be greeted by a golden retriever who is happy to see you is, usually lowers the anxiety level quite quickly. . . . So I think there is just the general sense of well-being and comfort the animal creates. I have had quite a few people identify a sense of safety when an animal is present. So safety I think is one element; emotional safety is another element."*

* * * * *

> *"It once again shows the comfort level and when it's quiet and relaxed, and pretty soon [Lucky]'s purring and we're more relaxed. They can take their time, and it might not feel as rushed to get to what we need to get to. And I think clients are more likely to stay with me longer and discuss their present issues of concern when he's here as well. . . . . The kids will want to stay longer."*

The participants spoke of the animal's "*presence being therapy in itself.*" The pets make the setting more natural. Even simple acts, such as caring for the animal's need for elimination, make the clients feel less inhibited: "*They'll ask if [Lucky] wants to use the litter box. I often thought whether kids would be like grossed out if he had to use like the litter box in here, but it hasn't fazed them at all.*"

Clients are calmer during sessions, from what was called a "*grounding*" effect of the animals. The dogs and cat also helped to meet a human need involving our connection to nature. One participant explained,

> *"My belief is that we used [to] . . . have animals around, and they used to be actively involved in the course of our lives. . . . We have progressively had less and less direct contact with animals in our society when I don't think psychologically we are prepared to have less and less contact. . . . I think that having an animal that's just present and free and responds completely of their own volition strikes something much more elemental in*

us as people that we have missing in our society. I think that what we do is we actually create more of a normal environment."

Unconditional Acceptance

The participants felt the companion animal's ability to provide unconditional acceptance and empathy played an important role during session. It was brought up fifty-nine times during the interviews. One psychologist attempted to explain this: *"I think the Rogerians would call it an unconditional positive regard. I think animals just have an innate capacity. . . ."* One participant stressed the animal's ability to be so genuine. When asked why he thought that occurred, he replied, *"No matter what. . . . The dog pretty much maintains that . . . unconditional positive regard."* Another replied, *"Pets, of course, are full of that unconditional positive regard."* One participant also spoke of the unconditional love supplied by an animal in the therapeutic setting:

"[Lucky] isn't going to call him a fatso or make fun of the fact that he's had chronic enuresis. And [the cat], he just loves this little boy. Like [Lucky] runs to him right away and sits on him and purrs on him and kneads and sleeps on him and plays with him. That's extremely positive. So what he might not be getting at the house, he'll get that unconditional, positive love at least with [the cat]. So I think that's excellent."

The participants, provided examples of the animals reacting intuitively to comfort clients. As one psychologist stated, *"[when] the kids are in an upset mood, he'll just sit quietly with them and purr. . . . It's amazing!"* When this psychologist was asked if animals did indeed have intuitive skills, the reply was, *"why do dogs seek out people in the middle of a waiting room to sit down [beside them]?"* Participants discussed their sense that the companion animal had an inborn sensitivity to the feelings of their clients. One stated, *"I do sense animals have a capacity to pick up on certain vibes, certain nonverbal vibes, and like [Digger] and [Cloey] are very good at reacting to that."*

One psychologist spoke of a touching scene when a child was hurting and the dog took it upon himself to comfort her. The dog went to her on his own, seeming to know the child needed the warmth and love he could provide.

"One of my clients was on the . . . comfy-cushion [a large bean bag] . . . talking about something that's painful . . . lying in kind of a manner that's kind

of like, kind of a crescent, and the dog will kind of crawl right up and crescent with her. It's like the dog's trying to absorb . . . that energy that's being transmitted by the client. So I was like, 'Wow!, That's quite interesting.' I didn't tell [Digger] to go there and neither did [the handler]. So it's quite powerful."

Nurturing

In the theme of enhanced environment, the animal's ability to supply the ingredient of nurturing was mentioned 215 times, which gave the impression it is a very prominent role for the animals during the therapeutic encounter. The animals not only supply nurture, they also teach about nurturing, and provide reciprocity in that they allow the client to nurture.

One participant told how he provides experiences throughout therapy to show nurturing behaviors:

"I will often give treats to him [dog] or have my clients give treats. . . . It . . . gives the message that beings are nurtured here . . . as you give nurture to [Bobby] you're also getting nurtured by his affection and attention back. I think that's very valuable for that sense of meeting needs. An animal's needs are simple, but they're straightforward enough in front, and when people are around and see those needs attended to — I think it helps a lot in knowing that their needs are going to be met when they come."

Many clients have not experienced caring relationships, so to see how one might treat another with kindness and love is powerful. One participant explains,

"When [Lucky] gets off the couch from where they're [the client and cat] sitting, you know, I will cuddle him or pet him or talk to him nicely. You know the kids are observing that. And do these kids need to be nurtured and are they missing that piece? Oh my gosh, yes!! So would they see me as someone who could provide that? Possibly yes . . . especially since many of the issues are abuse, neglect, abandonment. So they see someone caring for this other being . . . speaking nicely, offering praise. When need be, intervening. . . . So yeah, I think that's definitely a good thing for them to see."

Each spoke of the ethical guidelines that prevent them from being able to supply the physical contact many clients crave and need. They emphasized how the companion animal supplies the human need for touch by mentioning it fifty-eight times within this theme. As one participant explained,

> "I don't like to touch . . . what I'm willing to do – if there was no animal-assisted therapy – if clients are crying, my form of like affection, touch, is transferring tissue onto the client. 'Here, I care, but. . . .' When I can't provide that, that's what [Digger] can do. And so we do very well. We provide that outlet for touch, for that nurturing. Because of . . . ethical issues . . . you're never supposed to show that kind of affection . . . it creates a lot of problems for clients. . . . So [Digger] and [Cloey] just provide that . . . they can communicate that through therapy – you know just the expression of allowing for the person to make that contact – that tactile touch that facilitates that nurturing. That care and support."

Participants also spoke of the reciprocity that occurred when clients, who are nurtured by the companion animal, return the gentle care; "*I will say, watching a client brush [Lucky] gently or peacefully . . . provides an atmosphere of relaxation and calm and peace for everyone in the room.*"

This participant discussed how important the role of companion animals is in allowing clients to show affection:

> "I think people having the chance to show affection and have affection returned is a really important role. And of course, as I need to maintain my boundaries – where a person needs to give and receive affection, I have to of course be very clear. I can show affection in some ways, but I have to make sure that that never is at all dangerous in terms of crossing a professional boundary. But [Bobby] doesn't have any problem with that. So I think that giving and receiving affection is certainly an important role that he can play."

One participant also works at a military base and discussed the importance of his companion animal's role within this environment.

> "one of his big roles right now – I'm at the military base and there's all sorts of female medics that are in the medical facility that I work out of, and he gives people the chance to show affection. The military environment is a very utilitarian functional environment, not attending to anything other than the functional needs."

In another case, a participant spoke of an adolescent boy who had been very withdrawn and resistant during his sessions. To his surprise, this young boy was actually full of love to give. Had the animal never been present, this psychologist would not have known about the affection this boy so desperately needed to share. In providing this child with a living being he could reach out to, the psychologist became aware of an aspect of this boy about which he had not been aware.

> *"And the circumstances that involved his removal from the home was very traumatic for him. And so, he had all this energy, all this emotional energy to give and he had no one to give it to. . . . So seeing him pour out all the affection for the dog was very significant for me. It's almost [pause] he unleashed all this tension. And that was the impetus for him to open up."*

The companion animal also serves as a soothing object of affection; capable of supplying a tactile sense of connection for clients. The pets were cuddled, stroked, held, hugged, and kissed by all age groups of clients. One psychologist said, *"It's like she was able to connect with the animal. . . . [Cloey] was this object of affection for this client."*

> *"I worked with a young woman who had been sexually assaulted by a health care professional and was traumatized as a result of that and was referred to me for therapy, which was difficult because I'm a male. . . . One day when she came she was tearful – so tearful she could hardly speak. But she was very attached to [Bobby], and [Bobby] and she came into this office . . . she slipped off the sofa and sat beside him and petted him for about 20 minutes. And after she had calmed herself in petting him, then she could start to talk, and she needed to talk about. . . . So she was able to talk given that she had calmed herself. And then she said, [Psychologist], I couldn't be here if [Bobby] wasn't here. She said that he made her feel safe – that nothing bad was going to happen. And so he was certainly worth his weight in gold that day.*

An animal's presence is also helpful in maintaining a safe and nurturing environment when the psychologist is focused on more technical work. One participant explains,

> *"I think that one of the values [Bobby] adds is a sense of humanity to the environment. And sometimes some of the work that I am doing is more technical and if I'm having to assess – I try to stay away from all the dehumanizing practices of questionnaires and those sorts of things, but – I think there is a sense that – of more human; a warmer sense. I think he adds that presence."*

Clients form bonds with the companion animals. This positive relationship allows them to feel okay about themselves. A young boy who was in residential care had difficulty making friends with the other residents. The therapy animal became his friend.

"When he comes in, it's nice for him, because he calls [Lucky] my friend, my buddy, and he doesn't have any strong attachments to the kids within his house because he is being bullied. So perhaps this fills a type of companionship need when he comes and sees [Lucky]."

Creativity

The companion animals' enhancing creativity throughout the therapeutic process was mentioned twenty-five times. An important aspect of this fertile addition was the sense of play the companion animals brought to the therapy session. The sessions would also contain laughter brought on through the antics of the animal, who participants believed seemed to know instinctively just when to lighten up the atmosphere. *"It makes coming to therapy a less threatening environment because it's not completely talking. They might pause for a moment and brush him, or play with him, or talk to him, or absolutely nothing."* Another participant explains the importance of the playful aspect of animal-assisted therapy,

"For some of the children who come . . . children who come here I think he's really important because they get to . . . he can be playful and he can be . . . again, the nurturing, . . . and we show him tricks . . . creates a playful environment."

The animals were helpful at moving clients into activities involving the right brain. Participants could use the animals to stimulate the imagination of clients and to help them through the use of metaphors that included the pets. One of the companion animals even appears as a character in clients' trances during hypnosis:

"[Bobby] is often with me when I'm doing hypnosis and will often be snoring away during hypnosis and people will have included him in their trance. If I give them an image of walking along the beach, I will often hear that they were walking with [Bobby]. That's an interesting little intrusion."

THEME III: ENHANCED PROFESSIONAL PRACTICE

Adjunct Therapy

The companion animals were used as an adjunct therapy. The participants in this study felt it augmented treatment within the theoretical frameworks they followed. This included cognitive behavioral therapy, person-centered therapy, narrative therapy, interpersonal therapy, and work within the realm of marriage and family therapy. In total, reference to animal-assisted therapy being integrated into their form of therapies was mentioned 118 times.

Two of the participants practiced cognitive behavioral therapy and followed guidelines incorporating the animals into their treatment plans that were developed by The Chimo Project. An example can be seen in this participant's statement:

> "I love how it fits in with CBT [cognitive behavioral therapy]. I love being able to encourage kids to develop coping thoughts for the animal first and then for themselves. I love asking the question, 'Well, what would [Lucky] say to that?' 'What do you think [Lucky] would think if you did that?' 'How would [Lucky] feel if you decided to AWOL?'"

The animal can also teach positive behavior by showing their discomfort at having their boundaries intruded on.

> "a boy who had a tremendous amount of neglect since early childhood . . . extremely, extremely, abused. . . . I can personally say that I had my reservations on seeing this boy. He was very – for lack of a better term, very uninhibited . . . animal-assisted therapy is great in teaching boundaries to a client. I would have [Digger] come in session, and this boy would be all over him. . . . [Digger] enjoyed it. But the funniest thing . . . [Digger] was, 'WOW, easy there buddy. . . .' [Digger] was like trying to tell this boy, 'Hey.' And so when [Digger] backed away I told the boy, 'You see what [Digger] is doing? You know he's not usually like this, but I notice he's kind of backing away. What do you think is happening here?' Throughout that conversation he was able to learn a little about, you know, give him a little pet, but give a little space too."

One of the participants uses her cat to teach boundaries with children who have histories of sexual abuse.

> *"he [the cat] likes to knead on people with his paws and when he kneads he often goes for fleshy parts. So . . . that's okay with us, but for kids who've had abuse in their past or whose boundaries have been violated, it's an excellent opportunity to — for them to be assertive. . . . I suggest to them, 'Okay, if he's in your personal space or bubble, then what are you going to do about it?' So for example they say, 'No, I don't like that!' and they would move him."*

Animals are able to model empathy and also reach clients who have difficulty connecting with what others are feeling. One psychologist told the story of a young boy who had never shown empathy toward anyone else in the past. The therapy dog was unable to make an appointment because he was sick and needed to be taken to the vet.

> *"So . . . of course he's very disappointed. I was expecting that. But one thing I didn't expect was the boy to take some initiative in trying to say, 'Well, [Digger]'s not feeling well. We need to do something. Let's make him a get well card.' I'm like, 'That's a great idea. Let's do it.' So I helped him. . . . Never, had I ever done anything [artsy] in session. I've always asked him to draw pictures of some of his feelings, but I've never helped him. I've never seen this boy take the initiative to see and to invest some emotional investment. . . . He got all the kids in the class to sign the get well card for [Digger]. So it was really positive, and it was really good, and I was very proud that a boy with this much dysfunction, exposure, and deficits in his life, [that he] was able to do that. . . . I'd say the younger version of him, when I first had him in session, would have been, 'Ah! Darn! I don't want to see [Digger] again!' So, not so much connected to his own self, but there's a concern, there's even empathy, feelings of genuine concern."*

He stressed the difference the animal had made in this young boy's progress:

> *"Do you see any improvements, you know, when you teach a kid social skills? Is there learning? Can you apply that to a situation? With this one kid I can say yes. He was . . . one of things we're trying to teach a lot of our kids . . . feelings of empathy . . . or the consequence, knowing."*

Participants also used the animals in teaching clients through analogy. One participant in particular used this technique a lot to reach the adolescents he worked with. He spoke of a young girl who often put

The Role of Companion Animals in Counseling and Psychology

other children at risk by taking them with her when she would go "AWOL" from the residential facility. He had her play a game of fetch with the therapy dog that the young girl adored. He then asked her to pretend she was throwing the ball onto the freeway for the dog to retrieve. This is how the scenario ended:

> *"She hesitates. And I go good, let's go back inside. . . . Now, '[client], would you have thrown that ball? [Cloey] really trusts you, would put all her faith in you. Would you throw that ball out into the traffic?' And she goes, 'NO.' 'Well, why?' '[Cloey] will get killed.' And I'm like, 'Yeah, that's right, probably right. So isn't some of the behaviors you're doing in the house kind of similar? I mean you're taking kids that seem to trust you and seem to like you, you're taking them AWOL — you're out in the dangerous, dangerous environment. . . . So do you understand what I'm trying to illustrate?' And she's like, 'Yeah. I do.' My intent is that she takes this analogy, she'll remember the game of fetch, and maybe she can apply that."*

The animals play a role in assisting the psychologists to teach and practice various concepts. This was mentioned eighty-six times during the interviews. One participant explained that he initially thought animals would simply enhance the therapeutic environment. However,

> *"to my surprise, my pleasant surprise, is that it leads to other things as well. . . . I found it very useful that animal-assisted therapy could also be used as a teaching tool in helping to explore things such as social skills — teach social skills, learn about things that maybe they were never taught much, things like boundary issues. So it's a very instrumental tool in teaching things like social skills/life skills. And maybe an emotional regulation [tool]. And so a lot of these techniques were very strong — very impactful for me."*

One participant uses her cat to teach relaxation exercises,

> *"I've even used [Lucky] to do, like, belly breathing with the kids which of course is a component of CBT to help them reduce their anxiety. Cats breathe so nice and slow and they're relaxed, especially when they're purring, and it's a good tool I think, because if they don't have the cognitive ability to use their imagination. . . . They can just do their breathing in time with the cat, be relaxed and peaceful. . . . I think he allows for that safety to be built in there as well."*

The participants spoke of the animals enabling them to role-model in areas such as nurturing, discipline, behavior modification, and patience. The animals also allowed the clients to see the "softer" and "lighter" side of their psychologists through humor and play. One therapist talked of how dealing with the cat's inappropriate behavior at times can be a wonderful learning opportunity for the children she works with.

> *"Occasionally he [the cat] does get quite playful and frisky. . . . So at that time . . . it would be an opportunity for me to model how to address that behavior. We take him off and we engage him in an appropriate play behavior, so then the kids can see that as well. And then, also, he provides the opportunity for me to say, 'I like it when you do this [Lucky]' as opposed to 'bad.' I think we would call it like a differential reinforcement about our behaviors right?"*

The animals can also be incorporated into role-play scenarios during sessions. For example,

> *"They might not be able to, for example, role-play with me what they're going to say to their father who may be dying of cancer, or who's abandoning them, but they can sit and tell [Lucky] what they're going to say."*

One psychologist involved in this study did not use cognitive behavioral techniques. He preferred a more interpersonal framework. He stated that the animal's presence can also be seen as a therapeutic tool:

> *"I know that some of the other therapists in the Chimo project have done more structured things with them [the animals] – you know, like getting the kids to whisper the secrets to the dog, or using the dog as an object lesson. [Bobby] is more of just a 'presence,' and I use him much more just in terms of what his natural responses are rather than me working at engineering a particular role for him. . . . I think the sense of presence stuff – he's gone to sleep here – and you can still feel him.*

He later added, *". . . I don't think [Bobby] takes any value away. [Bobby] lets me do my job and doesn't interfere with that. So I think if any, there's added value."*

Clients do not tire of animal-assisted therapy and participants felt it did not lose its effect over time. One psychologist spoke of his experience:

"Some clients will respond well to art therapy. Some will respond well to play therapy, but one thing I do notice is . . . sometimes the therapeutic technique loses its novelty. But . . . I've had clients for quite some time and . . . they all enjoy having animal-assisted therapy. . . . They don't seem to tire of it. They always seem to appreciate the quality time that we spend."

Participants commented that the animal acts as an emotional indicator in regard to the clients. One participant talked of his dog's ability to alert him when clients are in distress. *"If [Bobby] is troubled in a session he will come beside me and hold up a paw for me to hold. He does it unobtrusively, so you know the client probably never knows, but it's [Bobby] saying something is going on here."* This participant told a story about a client who arrived early for an appointment:

". . . I just knew he was there early and I sent [Bobby] out to be with him until I could get my charting done so I could see him at one. And [Bobby] went out to him and then came back and looked at me through the open doorway, and looked at the client in the waiting room, and looked at me, and looked at the client. So I'm wondering 'What's going on here?' So I went out and I greeted him and he was in a lot of distress. I said to him, '[Client], do you want to come in?' and he said, 'Yes, I think I'd better.' . . . he said that when he came he was so agitated inside that it was all he could do to keep from picking up the coffee table and heaving it through the window. And then [Bobby] came and he felt better. But I'm sure [Bobby] was thinking, 'Wow, this is pretty heavy. I think I better get [the psychologist] for this one.' And so [Bobby] came and got me. . . . It is amazing. And [the client], I don't think read that [Bobby] was troubled, but [Bobby] read that [the client] was troubled and came. And I was able then to sit with [the client], of course and [Bobby] sit with him too, and talk with him."

The companion animals were referred to as cotherapist or working partners. Participants emphasized that the animals truly work along side them. *"[Lucky] in a sense is my cotherapist, and if I make a cat a cotherapist so to speak, that's me acknowledging the fact that there's more going on here than just him sitting and purring. There's actual work being done."*

Asset to Therapist's Well-Being

One aspect of the interview findings that I had not expected was the positive effect the animals had on the psychologists' sense of well-being. They each spoke of how much they gained from having the animal present, mentioning the contribution of the animal to their well-being thirty-five times. The two participants who brought their own pets seemed to understand their animals fed them emotionally and spiritually. As one psychologist put it, *"Part of me wanted to have an animal around for my own mental health."* Another psychologist stated:

> *"he's an, actually a joy and a treat for me to bring to work for my own self . . . an at-work perk . . . it's beneficial for the client – let me say that it's beneficial for me to have him at work. I'm typing up doing reports at the computer, and he's sitting on my lap purring. How nice is that? So that puts me, of course, in a more relaxed frame of mind, and I think I probably do better work, and I think I'm more productive."*

One psychologist who works within a group in private practice mentioned that his dog fits in well with all the therapists working at his office and enhances the environment of the entire office. Clients belonging to other psychologists often want [Bobby] to join them in session: *"If I came in . . . the door, [the other psychologist] would open the door so [Bobby] could go into the session."*

THEME IV: CREATING A SENSE OF SACREDNESS

Participants spoke of being aware of an invisible, intangible "essence" that seemed present when the dogs and cat were around. Each was aware that somehow this essence impacted and influenced their surroundings and their therapy. Words contained within this theme arose in their conversations a total of seventy-six times.

> *"There's something so peaceful that even I am seeing and feeling that there is peace and calm within this room. There's one client who's so gentle, she touches his ears so gentle and whiskers and face . . . he's like, 'yeah, whatever, this feels nice.' And she knows that it feels nice for him. And I'm watching her gently do this too. It's so peaceful and calming. There's definitely something. It affects us all in the room when that happens."*

Each participant spoke of this sense of peacefulness in the room when the animals are present. One said, *"It's like a warm nurturing environment that just totally envelops you and just heightens feelings of safety and trust." "And there are some really misty-eyed moments. I wouldn't give it up. .*

. . In a lot of ways it's very rewarding, it's a nice reward to have. . . . There's laughs, there's sometimes tears. It's a very powerful tool to have."

As I listened to their narratives, I frequently envisioned severely wounded children and adults clinging to a companion animal for comfort as they opened up in trust to finally tell their painful stories. I envisioned the Creator working through the animals, reaching out to people who had, in many cases, lost trust in humans. One participant pointed out that he was only able to help a severely traumatized young woman because of a dog:

> *"Well, I would not have been able to do the therapy with her without the dog in the room. Her dog was absolutely needed for things to be safe . . . this girl had no trust of social workers and psychologists at all. But, because I could speak dog, she could come here. So, what an important role for the animal to play!"*

One participant described the sense of sacredness that arises when witnessing the companion animal's empathy and sensitivity:

> *"I can remember one client just weeping, sitting on the sofa, and she was talking about the abuse that she had been a part of in the past, and her relationship with family members. And I just remember he [the cat] went right up to her and was laying his head right on her chest. He doesn't even do that at home with me. But it was pretty unbelievable. So there are sacred and powerful experiences that occur when the animal is present for sure."*

Another participant spoke of the dogs he worked with being able to "*bring the soul to feeling.*" He stated,

> *"I'm very envious of [Digger] and [Cloey]. I wish I could do that, but I'm a man, a male. . . . And so as warm and therapeutic and unconditional that I try to be to these kids, I'm just another authority figure. But not [Digger] or [Cloey]. They don't apply."*

Each of the excerpts on the companion animals acting as catalysts for healing could also be viewed within the framework of this theme. Although they spoke of it in different ways, in each participant, I could hear the awe and wonder they felt and their attempts to describe this sacred essence that supported their healing efforts.

"the animal's presence just increases that sensation – healing. But I think

. . . animal-assisted therapy is just including an animal – allowing the animal to be totally their own animate self and just allowing that to be part of the context for the client's healing."

One of the most striking aspects of the interviews was the number of times a participant could not find words to explain what he or she had witnessed. They could not explain the unexplainable, the mystery. Words such as amazing, awesome, unbelievable, wow, powerful, brilliant, surprising, wonderful, impactful, right on, positive, helpful and interesting, were used a total of fifty-one times.

I was struck by their sense of passion as the participants spoke of their experiences of working with a companion animal during therapy sessions and their sense of awe over the healing relationship between pet and the client.

Psychology tends to ignore what cannot be explained through empirical evidence. Yet, as one participant noted, *"You could interpret it in a number of ways. And you do find that as a sacred moment psychology would say, 'Oh great, anxiety reduction.' . . . As long as it's helping."*

During one interview, after an extremely moving story, I mentioned that I often feel the love of God coming through the eyes of a gentle dog. The participant responded, *"Absolutely! That is why God is dog spelled backward."*

Chapter 5

GNAWING ON THE RAWHIDE

As stated earlier, the purpose of this book was twofold. The first was to determine the role companion animals play in the process of counseling and psychology. The second was to apply the information gleaned to Winnicott's concept of the holding environment and transitional phenomena, which were formed through his understanding and use of object relations psychoanalytic theory.

As presented in Chapter 4, four major themes were extracted from the data collected for this study. These themes were (1) enhanced therapeutic alliance/relationship, (2) enhanced therapeutic environment, (3) enhanced professional practice, and (4) creating a sense of sacredness.

In this chapter, the themes and the subthemes that arose from the findings will be discussed and applied to Winnicott's concepts of the holding environment and transitional phenomena. Relevant literature will be presented in support of this discussion.

DESCRIPTION OF OBJECT RELATIONS THEORY AND WINNICOTT'S CONCEPTS

Object Relations Theory

Winnicott was a pediatrician who went on to study object relations psychoanalytic theory. He viewed the key aspect of healthy human development as rooted in relationships and microinteractions with people. Through applying this psychoanalytic theory to his work with mothers and their babies, he developed the concepts of the holding environment and transitional phenomena (Phillips, 1988).

Since Winnicott's theory base was that of object relations, it is important to have some understanding of the philosophical underpinnings of this theoretical framework. Object relations theory holds that the infant's experience in relationship with the mother, or primary caregiver, is the main determinant of personality formation. The infant's need for attachment to the primary caregiver is believed to be the motivating factor in the development of the infantile self (Scharff & Scharff, 1995).

According to this theory, humans are influenced the most by past and current relationships to other individuals as a main force for life. The need for an infant to bond with a primary caregiver is paramount and above the need for food, clothing, and shelter. External objects are those we relate to externally. An internal object may be a piece of psychic structure that influences the way we react to criticism, and another internal object may be a piece of psychic structure that influences the way we react to rejection. Each object has an affect that accompanies it (Cashdan, 1988).

In object relations theory, the treatment of clients is aimed at analyzing defenses, resistances, and transference, as well as dealing with such issues as shame, guilt and anxiety. Emphasis is placed on "making the unconscious conscious and bringing primary process material within secondary process organization" (Robbins, 1987, p. 66). According to Robbins, the ideal outcome of therapy involves "modifying the defenses of the ego and prohibitions of the superego, to allow the patient's life space to expand and to tolerate a richer symbolic and imaginative existence" (p. 66).

Robbins' thoughts are related to what one of the participants in this study experienced in his client's session when the animal is present, "I think that their [clients] general sense of well-being is enhanced. And so therefore, they're in an ego state or a mental, emotional state that they can more easily do work."

Winnicott's Concepts of the Holding Environment and Transitional Phenomena

In Winnicott's (1962) developmental theory, the infant is described as "unintegrated" for a good part of the time (as cited in Seinfeld, 1993, p. 103). The mother holds the infant, which provides a sense of wholeness to the child's sensory motor parts. "Winnicott's holding relationship [is] an expression of the maternal function that provides an authentic sense of being" (Seinfeld, 1993, p. 18).

Winnicott described two important aspects of relating in the mother-infant relationship. The first, the environmental mother, forms the context for the baby's growth and development. The mother provides an "arms-around" relationship, holding the baby and setting conditions for keeping the baby fed, clothed, warm and safe. She takes care of the physical and emotional environment for the infant (Scharff & Scharff, 1995).

For Winnicott, the earliest relationship of the baby to the mother is completely physical. According to Scharff and Scharff (1995), this completely physical relationship gives way to a progressively larger psychological relationship over the first few months of life. "It does so with the creation of what Winnicott called the potential space [or transitional space] between mother and baby" (p. 42).

Transitional phenomena, which represent the good-enough-mother, allow the baby to begin to separate from the symbiotic relation of the mother and child dyad. The *potential space* or *transitional space*, and the *transitional object*, are both transitional phenomena. The baby is able to enter the transitional space and begin to relate to the mother across a growing distance. Here the baby is free to discover what the mother is offering as though the baby had been the one to invent or create it. Also held within this transitional space are the baby's transitional objects, such as a favorite blanket. These objects belong to the baby entirely and are used, held, loved, and hated as the baby's own, and yet they represent the soothing and safety of the mother. By interacting with the transitional object, the baby can act as if it is in full control of its object mother (Kahane, 1993; Phillips, 1988; Scharff & Scharff, 1995; Winnicott, 1953).

In this transitional space, the baby is in communication with the holding environment provided by the mother (outer world), just as it is in communication with the direct object relations to the mother (inner world). It is this blend of the inner and outer world that provides the material of the baby's growing internal world. To Winnicott, this space was also the locus of creativity (Scharff & Scharff, 1995).

Within the envelope of this holding environment, the mother offers the baby a direct object relationship, which Winnicott referred to as the object mother. This mother is the object of the infant's love, hate, interest, and desire. "Within the envelope provided by the environmental mother, the baby is free to find itself. In the relationship with the mother as an object, the baby is provided with the stuff from which to build its own internal objects" (Scharff & Scharff, 1995, p. 42). Through the infant's experience with the environmental mother and the object mother, and between the whole mother and infant, the child develops its internalized object relationships and sense of self.

The therapeutic relationship offers a holding environment similar to that of the mother and infant dyad. Patterns can emerge, yet be different enough for identification and reworking. This is done through the therapist's capacity for "holding" the client, for sharing the client's experience, for tolerating the anxiety involved, and for providing transitional space where understanding can be cultivated (Scharff & Scharff, 1995). "The holding function frequently is represented by the [therapist's] ability to create a sense of emotional space with firm edges – a room large enough to allow for wide and intense affective expression, yet simultaneously bounded enough always to feel containing to the [client]" (Slochower, 1996, p. 23).

APPLICATION OF THEMES TO WINNICOTT'S "HOLDING ENVIRONMENT"

Theme of Enhanced Therapeutic Alliance/Relationship

Trust

The results demonstrated that companion animals may have increased the level of trust clients felt toward their psychologist. Trust is an important element in the holding environment. The client has to have faith in the ability of the therapist to "hold them" psychologically during times when they are overwhelmed with intense feelings. This participant discussed how a "very defensive" client "warmed" up to the therapist through the animal's presence. "With the addition of [Cloey] the client was . . . very engaged in the session; was very 'on' – had very positive feelings. And I noticed another thing. . . . I would notice the warmth the client would generalize towards me." Another therapist explained, "We're going to talk about things that are painful, that are uncomfortable – they're very reluctant to talk about. In a lot of ways it [animal-assisted therapy] facilitates a sense of trust." Could

80   *The Role of Companion Animals in Counseling and Psychology*

it be that the animals enhanced the sense of holding within the therapeutic environment?

Catalyst for Enhanced Healing

The results indicate that the animals may act as a catalyst for enhanced healing. The holding environment is a place where clients confront fears, and because enhanced healing was a notion frequently mentioned by the participants in this study, it would appear that the animals' presence was a catalyst, allowing for the clients' willingness to risk sharing personal information in order to discover and grow. One could wonder if the animals acted as the transitional phenomena of the good-enough-mother, allowing clients to feel secure enough in the holding environment to venture into the transitional space of the known and unknown.

Theme of Enhanced Therapeutic Environment

Warm, Friendly and Safe Environment

The results suggest that the animals provided a warm, friendly, and safe environment. Participants emphasized the profound positive changes that seemed to occur with the addition of the companion animal. The companion animal appeared to supply the needed ingredients to make the therapeutic encounter occur in a less threatening atmosphere. Buckley (1986) and Pine (1984) have suggested that central to the holding environment as a precondition for conducting supportive therapy, the therapist must ensure the "safety" of the therapeutic environment. The participants often mentioned what they believed was an increase in the clients' sense of safety.

Dr. Constance Perin first suggested that a pet could be the symbolic equivalent of the mother in 1980. She felt the mother-child symbiotic relationship of complete devotion resembles a dog's "complete and total love," "utter devotion," and "life-long fidelity." She stated, "Speechless, yet communicating perfectly, the mute and ever-attentive dog is a symbol of our own memory of the magical once-in-a-lifetime bond" (as cited in Beck & Katcher, 1996, pp. 68–69).

In being "mothered by the pet," Perin has suggested a person is able to recreate the faith of the infant in superabundant love. Beck and Katcher (1996) agreed with her, stating, "Precisely because pets have the ability to recreate a mythic love for self, they can be used to requite love when human love has failed" (p. 73). Could it be this "mothering" by the pet represents both the environmental mother and the object mother discussed earlier? Could the pet represent the phenomena of the good-enough-mother?

Unconditional Acceptance

As discussed in Chapter 4, there was also considerable evidence to indicate that animals in therapy sessions provide unconditional acceptance. Many involved in the field of animal-assisted therapy have stated that pets, especially dogs, seem to possess several of the characteristics that Carl Rogers (1951, 1961, 1989) and Robert Carkhuff (1969, Truax & Carkhuff, 1967) described as being so important to the therapeutic relationship (Katcher, 1981; Kruger & Serpell, 2006; Parshall, 2003; Ruckert, 1987). These were unconditional positive regard, genuineness, congruence between experience and expression, and a capacity for empathy. These qualities must also be present in order to create a holding environment for clients (Ashbrook, 1996). The results documented in this book suggest the companion animals may possess these necessary qualities.

The pastoral theologian Charles W. Taylor (1991) combined all of the identified basic features of therapeutic facilitation into the single idea of "presence." It would seem that Taylor's definition of presence coincides with what the participants in this study believe the animals bring to the therapeutic encounter. As I reflected on this possibility in reference to the themes that arose from the interviews, I wondered whether the animal's presence could play a role in supporting a therapist's presence and, therefore, assist in the creation and maintenance of a holding environment for clients.

Corson and Corson (1980) referred to pets as "nonverbal communication mediators" and claimed they offered "a form of nonthreatening, nonjudgmental, reassuring nonverbal communication and tactile comfort and thus helped to break the vicious cycle of loneliness, helplessness and social withdrawal" (p. 107). This was also a belief held by the participants.

Levinson (1969) supported the view expressed by Berl (1952), who emphasized that emotionally disturbed individuals who have experienced difficulty in their relationships with people relate more easily or quickly to animals. Levinson believed that animals offered nonthreatening, nonjudgmental, and essential unconditional attention and affection. Could the animals provide the acceptance that could help open "emotionally disturbed" clients to the acceptance of the therapist? Participants in the project believed this was so, indicating that the animals acted as a bridge, allowing them to connect with clients.

Participants described how the animals in their therapeutic settings offered emotional responsiveness, which facilitated the process of empathy. Many of the clients seen by the participants experienced a poor mother-child relationship, which meant they struggled with the absence of a central figure to give cohesion to their life. As Robbins (1987) reminds us, cognitive awareness is of little help. The client needs a relationship in treatment that would "both repair the damages of loss and give him or her courage to live through her [or his] feelings of pain and abandonment" (p. 67).

The results offered evidence that the animals supply "mirroring" or "resonance," which is part of the mother's role in the holding environment. Issues commonly encountered when dealing with primitive mental states involve the loss of boundaries and regression to fusion states. Both of these are tested out and experienced within the treatment relationship. The results of this project indicated that the companion animals involved seemed to help mirror internal object relations and contain emotions while clients dealt with their associated defenses and developmental problems. Examples, such as the cat placing its head on the chest of a client as she wept or the dog crawling up beside a client and curling in to "crescent with her," were provided in Chapter 4.

As I reviewed the collected information and extracted themes I wondered whether the animal could be attempting to contain or hold the intense emotions for this client. Were the animals representing both the good-enough-mother and the environmental mother discussed earlier? Evidence seemed to indicate that this is true. These questions will now be discussed in greater detail.

Nurturing

Participants in this project felt the animal's presence was a source of nurturing to the clients, providing them with a sense of caring, calming, and comforting. Participants believed their clients had lower levels of anxiety, and the animals acted to soothe clients through the tactile comfort of their soft, warm bodies. Participants found the animals were important in meeting the need for touch in all of their clients, but especially in adolescent boys and clients in the military, for whom displays of affection between people are not seen as acceptable.

Participants spoke of the animals being petted, stroked, hugged, kissed, and held. Winnicott usually met the client's touch needs in the form of hand or head holding (Seinfeld, 1993). Spitz (1946), Harlow (1959), Bowlby (1973), and Harper (1994) and numerous others have empirically demonstrated the human need for touch, and its relationship to physical, mental, emotional, and spiritual well-being.

Each of the participants stressed how much they appreciated having an animal present as a form of tactile comfort for clients and as a means for clients to give and receive affection. They each spoke of the ethical issues governing the profession, and the need to remain vigilant over maintaining proper boundaries. One participant stated, "*I'm very cognizant of how vulnerable not just the client is, but the vulnerable [position] that I can put myself into.*" When the dog is present, this participant can say, "*Let those feelings go. Hug [Digger] as much as you want.*" How wonderful it is that touch can be ethically included in the holding environment through companion animals!

Creativity

Therapeutic play facilitates the creation of a holding environment of relatedness and resonance (Winnicott, 1953). The discoveries contained within this book indicate the animals acted to enhance safety and creativity (play), which means they facilitated the creation of a holding environment. Much like a toddler who needs to feel safe before he can lose himself in play, the client must feel safe in order to do the same. In this "in between" space of creativity, the client and the therapist can take on assigned roles and act them out much like a child will take on roles when playing.

Winnicott (1953) believed therapy was play, and it was through play that a client transitioned into a new level of self-awareness. The results indicating that the animals seemed to act as a catalyst for growth and increased self-awareness could also imply that the animals enhanced clients' abilities to work within the holding environment, where play and creativity occur in the transitional space.

Theme of Enhanced Professional Practice

Adjunct Therapy

As mentioned previously, there was evidence to indicate that the animals serve as an adjunct form of therapy. Fine and Mio (2006) believe it is important for the general community to recognize that there is a difference in the services rendered through animal-assisted activities and those through animal-assisted therapy. Much of the literature on animal-assisted therapy focuses on activities done with or through the companion animal. Participants used both animal-assisted activity and animal-assisted therapy, and believed the animals' presence was therapy in itself.

When the therapy animals are not involved in activities, they are considered to be visiting with or interacting (Wilson, 2006). One of the participants used pets as an adjunct therapy in structured cognitive behavioral activities but also believed the animals' presence is a form of therapy in and of itself. Another used therapy dogs in structured cognitive behavioral activities but also practiced person-centered therapy. He emphasized the animals' ability to provide "unconditional positive regard" and stated, "just their presence, being here is therapy in itself."

A third participant, who does not practice cognitive behavioral therapy but practices narrative therapy integrated with interpersonal therapy as well as marital and family systems therapy, believes the animal creates "a healing context" simply by being present in the room. The results of this project appear to demonstrate that the animal's presence and interaction with clients could be used in conjunction with many theoretical frameworks because all the participants believed the animals' presence was therapeutic. As stated earlier, Ashbrook (1996) believed this presence was needed to create a holding environment for clients.

The animals seemed to "hold" the clients at times when the therapist was unable to do so. One participant mentioned that "*sometimes some of the work that I am doing is more technical.*" He explained that one of the "*values [Bobby] adds is a sense of humanity . . . more human; a warmer sense.*" Another participant said that at times, "*I just kind of facilitate the therapeutic warmth and regard. Once in a while I interject with concepts. So when they're in that positive space, in that comfortable setting, it's not like I'm prodding . . .*"

Gnawing on the Rawhide

In discussing the process of holding, Slochower (1996) mentions certain clients are "extremely sensitive to slights of any kind." Even breaking into a highly sensitive person's narrative can be experienced as so "assaultive that the [client] reacts with a sense of profound injury" (p. 65). In dependent clients, "even small alterations in the therapist's even responsiveness can be highly disturbing" (p. 73). These failures in holding can be expressed through stalls in the therapeutic process by way of defiance, withdrawn periods of silence, or even abrupt terminations of therapy.

The experience of safety is implicit in the holding process. In traumatized clients, a failure in the holding capacity of the therapist may represent a traumatic reenactment to the client and can even push a client toward a more defensive level of functioning. Yet, Slochower (1996) stated it is inevitable that a therapist's ability to maintain a holding stance will break down. A time of repair is then needed to rebuild the trust of the client. The findings in this study indicate that a companion animal may be able to maintain the holding environment for the therapist during these "breakdowns," thus possibly eliminating the need for, or reducing the time for, repair.

Asset to the Therapist's Well-Being

Participants described feeling a higher sense of well-being when the animals were present and emphasized they considered the animals to act as cotherapists.

"I think I [muffled] better professionally registered psychologist when my animal is with me in the room and assisting the kids. And I think the kids are more open when they're here. I think there's obviously a comfort level . . ."

* * * * *

"I think there are advantages for me. . . . I think it's just a little bit of a sense of regrounding me."

* * * * *

"May I be so bold as to say that I find the therapy more productive, and the exercises more creative and really being more motivated to engage when the animal is present than if he is not present."

The ability of animals to enhance the working environment, while a surprise finding is consistent with the literature on pets' providing physiological benefits for the staff. Barker, Kniseley, McCain, and Best (2005) measured serum cortisol, epinephrine, norepinephrine, salivary cortisol, salivary immunoglobulin A, and blood for lymphocyte counts in twenty health care workers before and after interacting with a visiting therapy dog. It was discovered that stress reduction occurred within as little as five minutes of interaction with the animal.

The decrease in cortisol brought on by the visiting animals was similar to those that occur during twenty minutes of rest. If visiting pets can have such a positive effect on staff exposed to them for only a few minutes, it seems a likely conclusion that those working with a companion animal present during most their work with clients would feel an increased sense of well-being.

While discussing the impact of an animal's presence on work atmosphere and job satisfaction, Joachin (2001) stated, "our hunch is that a therapy animal program on premise also contributes to lower self-reports of employee stress and higher job satisfaction ratings" (p. 292). The results from this project agree with Joachin's "hunch." The presence of the animal brought a sense of comfort to the psychologists while they worked. They stated they felt more grounded, more relaxed, more productive, softer, and more creative. This positive effect on the participants could only serve to enhance the therapeutic encounter between client and therapist, and one could conclude such circumstance can only strengthen the therapist's ability to "hold" the client.

Theme of Creating a Sense of Sacredness

The cat and dogs involved in this project seemed to bring about a sense of the sacred. Participants spoke of the animal's presence bringing "peacefulness" and "connections to soul." After hearing many of the participants struggle to explain the "magical" effect the pets seemed to have on clients, I recognized they were attempting to explain the mystery of spirit. While there are no formal studies to be found on this topic, there are many anecdotal reports of how peoples' lives were improved by therapy pets and companion animals (Becker, 2002; Butler, 2004; Crawford & Pomerinke, 2003; Goldstein, 1999; Kowalski, 1999; McElroy, 1996; Nicoll, 2005; Randour, 2000; Schoen, 2001; Schoen & Proctor, 1995; Stone, 2002).

The sense of the sacred created by the participating animals seemed to enhance both the client's and therapist's ability to be "transcendent," meaning "that which goes beyond conscious control" (Ashbrook, 1996, p. 20). In transcending, we reach the limit of what we can do rationally and let go of the expectation that we can control. Safety replaces defense, and we respond more adaptively (Gilbert, 1989). Comments from the participants indicate this process takes place for them during therapy sessions when the animals are present.

The relationship between animal and human is void of judgment or labeling, so opportunities for increased awareness and new learnings are endless. One participant believed the constant "unconditional positive regard" supplied by animals worked to *"break down the natural defenses, the natural barriers, to allow them [clients] to disclose and share feelings."* As stated by Nicoll, "The power of healing offered by the human-animal bond can transcend us and connect us to our inner core, our soul" (2005, p. 41). As one participant stated, *"[Digger] . . . does wonderful work that just helps the soul to feelings regarding disclosure, emotional issues."*

In listing the benefits of animal-assisted therapy in their training manual, the Delta Society (2004) included what I believe to represent aspects of the results contained within the theme creating a sense of sacredness. They refer to a "something more" being supplied through the presence of animals and discuss how many have reported this to be "a spiritual fulfillment or a sense of oneness with life and nature" (p. 18). They also refer to author J. Allen Boone (1954/1976), who stated that his relationships with animals and nature are "part of [his] sustaining the energy and/or part of [his] communion and relationship with the divine" (Delta Society, 2004, p. 18).

Bekoff believed companion animals "offer important lessons in spirituality and can be catalysts in our weaving a seamless tapestry with all life in which the interconnections are rich, deep, and innumerable" (2001, p. 645). Through her experience working in animal-assisted therapy, Butler has come to view the work of a therapy dog as an intimate journey among the dog, the client and the therapist: "Working with therapy dogs is an ongoing process of self-assessment, reflection, and willingness to see another species as sometimes more capable and more compassionate than ourselves. By being open to the gifts of animals, we increase our own opportunities for growth" (2004, p. 14).

Ashbrook (1996) stated that our presence as a counselor or psychologist provides refuge from the "onslaught of worldly demands" in the sacred space of the therapeutic environment. He added, "Psychotherapists call this the 'holding environment'" (p. 12). In his point of view, the therapist's steadiness allows clients to "re-expose themselves to the harsh elements, to experiment with new life, to re-engage in living with others" (pp. 12–13). Evidence from this project indicates that the animals used in therapy by participants could also provide steadiness by anchoring or grounding clients in the safety of the holding environment. An example can be seen in this participant's comment: "*he will come . . . quite close to the person and he'll lay down and even lay on their feet as if to ground the person.*"

"Theologically, unconditional positive regard and empathic mirroring suggest agape, the Greed word for 'love'" (Ashbrook, 1996, p. 86). Ashbrook also stated that agape, which "involves an intentional and intelligent cherishing of others' well-being," is a prerequisite for a holding relationship (p. 86). Participants provided evidence supporting the notion that the therapy cat and dogs involved mirrored empathy and supplied clients with genuine unconditional positive regard. Could it be a sense of sacredness was created in part out of a pet's ability to supply agape? Could it be that this agape supports that of the therapist in creating a holding environment?

Bekoff (2001) believed dogs and other pet companions "engage us with the natural world and, indeed, with ourselves" (p. 645). Becker (2002) believes that the power animals hold, in emotionally charged situations, stems from their ability to speak the language of the soul. One could wonder whether or not the animals' presence could be viewed as a vehicle to assist people in feeling and experiencing the divine that dwells within their being, within others, and indeed, within all creation.

"There are many worlds beyond the human experience" (Bekoff, 2001, p. 643). Animals are meaningful to humans because they "act as a bridge to both the natural and supernatural" (Dresser, 2000). As stated by Michael Fox, a veterinarian since 1962, "Animals encourage us toward communion with the sacred dimension of reality that is as empowering and healing as it is inspiring and affirming" (as cited in McElroy, 1996, p. xvii).

Many believe our relationship with animals offers an extraordinary spiritual opportunity. The essence of spirituality can be explained in part as love; Buber (1996) wrote, "If you wish to believe, love!" (p. 136) (as cited in Randour, 2000, p. 58). All of the participants commented on how their animals showed clients love without reservation, judgment, or expectation; their love was "unconditional." They also observed the clients showing loving behaviors toward the animals. Could the animals' unconditional love open the clients to spirit by opening them up to love?

After examining all of the evidence and reviewing the literature on animal-assisted therapy, I conclude animals in a therapeutic setting act as catalysts in the holding environment, assisting clients to feel connected to spirit. Clients are able to experience the pure and accepting love of the Creator through the agape supplied by the presence of the pet, as they struggle through the wilderness of the unknown and the known in the transitional space. Jesus actually "prepared for his work by dwelling in the wilderness with the wild animals" (Mark 1:13) (Eaton, 1995, p. 112). As the "Tempter came with his wiles," Jesus was able to stand firm because the animals surrounded him "with their pure love" (p. 113). Perhaps the companion animals also enable clients to stand firm in the transitional space by surrounding them with the unconditional love, comfort and safety of the Creator as good-enough-mother within the holding environment.

APPLICATION OF THEMES TO WINNICOTT'S TRANSITIONAL PHENOMENA

The holding environment helps a client enter the transitional space by sheltering the person from becoming overwhelmed. In the holding environment, threat is contained from both the outer and the inner world (Ashbrook, 1996). The evidence contained within this book indicates that companion animals may play a role in facilitating the creation of Winnicott's (1953) twofold formulation of transitional phenomena, which act as agents of the good-enough-mother within the holding environment.

Transitional Space

Winnicott (1953) referred to the area between inner and outer worlds as the "transitional space." Noonan (1998) suggested that pets can be important mediators in the relationship to the transitional space. She believed the animal's ability to enhance transitional phenomena actually helps people achieve a "kind of wholeness" (p. 27). Numerous references in psychoanalytic literature address the clients' enhanced ability to reveal or discuss difficult thoughts, feelings, motivations, or conflicts when pets are present. It is also documented that clients project these same emotions onto the animal (Mason & Hagan, 1999; Reichert, 1998; Serpell, 2000b; Wells, Rosen, & Walshaw, 1997). An example of projective identification can be seen in the following excerpt:

> *"So for example if the presenting symptoms are anxiety. . . . Then I'd have them identify [Lucky]'s anxious thoughts and then I'd have them identify hope and thoughts for [Lucky]. And then I would get them to do that for themselves."*

All creative and spontaneous gestures are initiated within the transitional space (Phillips, 1988). This is where play occurs; in a virtual world that contains aspects of reality and aspects of the imagination. The suggestion by many authors that animals act as a mediator between the conscious and the unconscious (Serpell, 2000b) can be seen in the experience of one participant who practices hypnosis. He has noted that his dog [Bobby] often appears in the trances of his clients, "*I give them an image of walking along the beach; I will often hear that they were walking with [Bobby].*"

Play occurs in the transitional space, and Winnicott (1953) believed we grow and develop a greater sense of self through working in this space. In other words, we heal through play, and according to Winnicott, therapy is play. The results provided evidence that suggests animals enhance the playfulness of therapy. Could it be that what appeared to be enhanced creativity brought on by the animals could be related to Levinson's (1969) belief that pets provide clients with a relatively neutral medium through which to express unconscious emotional material? Both Levinson (1969) and Sarmicanic (2004) believed animals act as catalysts for self-reflection because they are imbued with qualities of the projected self.

It is in the transitional space that old feelings, thoughts, and behaviors are awakened for modification – in order to make a transition (Robbins, 1987; Winnicott, 1971/2005). Participants indicated the animals helped clients to make transitions by playing a role in projective identification; role play; metaphors; and analogy; imagery; and relaxation exercises.

The results of this project seemed to indicate that the animals unconsciously held the key to a client's inner self, allowing them to move through layers of masks and defenses. According to Davis & Juhasz (1995), pets increase a person's understanding of the world through their ability to supply a certain sense of empowerment that makes addressing fears more tolerable. The pet's presence seemed to bring into focus, in a totally instinctual way, what was felt and needed during moments of vulnerability in the client. This conclusion is in agreement with Kruger and Serpell (2006), who believe clients may achieve a greater sense of comfort in the working alliance through the animal's presence, which may in turn hasten compliance and retention in treatment as well as treatment outcomes.

In object relations theory, inner representations of one's past are expressed within the complex interaction of objective and subjective realities that create a psychological space (transitional space) between two people from the beginning of therapy. "Within this space, past and present merge to create a unique mood and atmosphere" (Robbins, 1987, p. 64). As indicated by the evidence, the companion animals seemed to bring the safety and comfort needed for clients to investigate and experience their object world within the transitional space. Clients seemed able to tolerate higher levels of discomfort when confronting sensitive topics.

Participants found that, clients often freely disclosed information regarding their past while playing with or stroking the pets. Animals seem to have the uncanny ability to help people recall memories (Fine, 2000). When the pets were present, participants noticed that clients often divulged themes of abuse, abandonment, and neglect, along with the internal conflicts causing their discomfort.

Through her work with at-risk children, Nicoll (2005) has come to understand that working with pets takes therapists into "unknown spaces." It is in these spaces where the creation of a relationship between client and animal provides the foundation for an intricate look at how clients function in other relationships. It is a "sacred negotiation of self-exploration, self-definition and self-reliance" that takes place in the present moment (p. 39). One could wonder if Nicoll's reference to "unknown spaces" represents Winnicott's (1953) concept of the transitional space.

The evidence provided suggests that companion animals may

enhance play. In Winnicott's opinion, both client and therapist must be prepared to play in order to recover early creativity and re-create the transitional space that is so necessary to bridge inner and outer realities. According to Winnicott, play is therapy and therapy is play or, in some cases, moving the client toward being able to play. Play was not aimless activity or simply having fun (Robbins, 1987).

> The essence of play in therapy involves the capacity to relax intellectual controls, and to become non-goal-oriented and open-ended in experiencing and working with the psychological space of the patients. Here images and symbols move into consciousness with their own logic and organization regarding time and place. Through symbolic play, patients are helped to organize psychological space. . . . Therapeutic play, then, becomes the means by which to create a holding environment of relatedness and resonance within which deficits in early object relations can be repaired and the potential for creative living can be regenerated (Robbins, 1987, p. 71).

Transitional Object

The transitional object is defined by Winnicott (1953) as an item or object, such as a blanket or soft toy, which serves a soothing function for a child. It is used to control the normal developmental stress of separation from the primary caregiver. The purpose of a transitional object is to act as a bridge to a higher and more socially acceptable level of functioning, not to serve as a substitute for failed or inadequate human relationships. As adults, individuals may not have completely separated and, thus, remain attached to various transitional objects. These offer a sense of security and can be in the form of photographs, religious paraphernalia, and other such articles that bring a sense of comfort.

Interaction with a trained companion animal during a session of therapy has been reported to reduce anxiety and serve as a source of comfort for the client (Barker & Dawson, 1998; Chimo Project Final Team Report, 2003; Shiloh, Sorek & Terkel, 2003). Through their studies on pets and humans, McNicholas & Collis (2006) concluded pets provide comfort (especially tactile comfort) and a sense of being cared for. They found the animals also enhanced the level of trust in clients which allowed for the release of emotions and feelings that subjects had felt unable to disclose to human sources of support. DeMello's (1999) study found that the anxiety-reducing effect of stroking a pet occurred independent of gender or general attitudes towards animals, as did the study by Shiloh and colleagues (2003). They stated, "the anxiety reducing effect of [animals] applied to people with different attitudes towards animals and was not restricted to animal lovers" (p. 387).

The findings of these empirically based studies are consistent with the evidence gleaned from the interviews with participants. Each noticed that clients appeared more relaxed when petting, stroking, cuddling, or holding a pet during their sessions. Because transitional objects are used to control anxiety, one could conclude that the animals in this study acted as transitional objects. This effect was earlier reported by Bachman & Bachman (2003), who stated that pets supplied unconditional love and acted like a "security blanket" during therapy, especially with children who have been abused or neglected (p. 2). This can be seen in the following example:

> *"And she had come in, and she said she had been crying when she came in, and [Bobby] sat in front of her and lifted a paw up for her to hold paws with him. And then when that paw got tired being held up he put it down and lifted the other front paw. And she said, 'We've just been going from one paw to another for the 20 minutes and I'm feeling so much better now.'"*

In 1970, Harold Bridger suggested that a companion animal is one maturational step beyond the transitional object. He felt that since an animal is alive and will walk away or "talk back," "it can occupy a place between the inanimate and animate which makes it a rich source of relating" (as cited in Noonan, 1998, p. 23). Other researchers since seem to agree with Bridger and add that animals are a more socially acceptable type of attachment object, rather than blankets and teddy bears, particularly among school-age children and adults (Perin, 1981; Serpell, 1993). Katcher (2000) suggested that animals acting as transitional objects be referred to as "transitional beings." Bridger's (1970) concept of animals acting as mature transitional objects during therapy and Katcher's (2000) suggestion that animals act as transitional beings are supported by the results of this project because there was reciprocity in the affection shown and the nurturing that occurred. Participants believed this reciprocity served to assist clients in the development of empathy and an understanding of nurturance.

Triebenbacher's (1998) study explored children's perceptions of the

94   *The Role of Companion Animals in Counseling and Psychology*

roles and functions of pets in their lives. She looked at areas such as comfort, security and emotional support. Her findings were (1) physical contact and ritualistic behaviors such as rubbing, hugging, and cuddling that are associated with inanimate transitional objects also occur between children and pets and (2) attachment behaviors such as proximity-seeking, initiating interactions, expression of affection, and thinking about the object of attachment also occurs in relation to pets and children. Participants in this project reported these same observations in relation to their clients and the animals.

The study by Triebenbacher (1998) supports the idea that companion animals offer emotional support, affection, and unconditional love in ways similar to transitional objects. This concurs with the statements of participants in this study. Clients seemed to form an attachment to the therapy animal that appeared to provide a sense of security, warmth, comfort, acceptance, and soothing during stressful periods in therapy,

> *"She would become quite anxious knowing the types of things she needs to work on. But when she walked through the door and saw [Bobby] . . . suddenly she felt okay; that she could do the work."*

An interesting discovery was that clients who did not seem to develop an attachment to the animals also seemed to have difficulty attaching to humans. As stated by one participant, "*It probably is a sign of the degree to which the child attaches to [Bobby]; is probably a sign in terms of their own attachment needs.*" Another participant expressed similar ideas when asked about clients who did not seem to bond with the animal: "*she wasn't connecting with identifying thoughts, behaviors, for [Lucky] and then herself . . . potentially she'd be a kid with difficulty attaching . . . probably so because she was a child who was abandoned by her mother, on and off.*"

CONCLUSION

The evidence collected from the participants suggests that the cat and dogs used as therapy animals in this study played a role in the creation and maintenance of what Winnicott referred to as "the holding environment" (Table 5-1). The participants reported that the animals seemed to enhance trust; act as catalysts for healing; provide a warm, friendly, safe environment, unconditional acceptance, empathy, nurturing, soothing and comfort through tactile connection; give and receive affection; and mirror internal object relations while assisting to contain the client's emotions.

The participants reported an enhanced sense of well-being with the animals present, which could possibly enhance the therapist's ability to hold the client. The results also indicate the animals may act to maintain the holding environment during "breakdowns" in the therapist's holding, thus perhaps decreasing or negating the time needed for repair.

In applying the results contained within the theme of *creating a sense of sacredness*, to Ashbrook's (1996) theological view of the holding environment, the animals appear to supply presence, agape, and an anchoring or grounding. The evidence also suggests that the animals may enhance the therapist's and the client's ability to "transcend."

The participating cat and dogs helped provide the trust and safety needed for clients to work within the transitional space. The animals were used in projective identification, role-play, metaphors, analogy, imagery, and relaxation exercises that could be seen as an indication of the cat and dogs facilitating the creativity needed for transitional work. Participants also noticed that clients seemed to freely disclose information about their past when the animals were present (Table 5-2).

Participants reported that clients were observed using the animals in ways that allow one to infer that they were being viewed as mature transitional objects (Bridger, 1970) or transitional beings (Katcher, 2000) (Table 5-2). Participants mentioned incidents in which the client-animal interactions involved physical contact. They observed clients performing ritualistic behaviors with the animals such as rubbing, hugging, kissing, holding, and cuddling, and they reported that clients appeared to display proximity-seeking behaviors, initiate interactions, express affection to the animals, and think about the object of attachment in and outside the therapeutic setting.

Table 5-1: Holding Environment

Enhanced Therapeutic Relationship	Enhanced Therapeutic Environment	Enhanced Professional Practice	Creating of a Sense of Sacredness
1. Animal's presence appeared to increase the level of trust clients felt toward their psychologist. 2. Animal's presence appeared to be a catalyst, allowing for the client's willingness to risk in order to discover and grow.	1. Animals provided a warm, friendly, and safe environment. 2. Clients had an increased sense of safety. 3. Animals provided unconditional acceptance. 4. Animals offered emotional responsiveness, which facilitated the process of empathy. 5. Animals supplied "mirroring" or "resonance," which is part of the mother's role in the holding environment. 6. Animals seemed to help mirror internal object relations and contain emotions while clients dealt with their associated defenses and developmental problems. 7. Animal's presence was a source of nurturing to the clients. 8. Clients had lower levels of anxiety. 9. Animals soothed clients through the tactile comfort. 10. Animals provided a form of tactile comfort for clients. 11. Animals were a means for clients to give and receive affection.	1. Animals' "presence" acted as an adjunct form of therapy. 2. Animals may have maintained the holding environment for the therapist during "breakdowns." 3. Animals may have reduced time to repair breakdown to minimal to none. 4. Animals may have enhanced participants' sense of well-being, and thus may enhance their ability to "hold" the client.	1. Animals may have enhanced client's and therapist's ability to "transcend." 2- Animal may have provided steadiness by anchoring or grounding. "agape" 3. Animals may have provided "agape," which could support that of the therapist's in creating a holding environment. 4. Animals provided "presence" through showing positive regard, genuineness, congruence, and a capacity for empathy.

Table 5-2: Transitional Phenomena

Themes	Transitional Space	Transitional Object
1. Enhanced Therapeutic Relationship 2. Enhanced Therapeutic Environment 3. Professional Practice 4. Creation of a Sense of Sacredness	1. Animals used in projective identification, role-play, metaphors, analogy, imagery, and relaxation exercises. 2. Animals facilitated a sense of trust; animals have ability to break down barriers. 3. Animals gave clients confidence and support to begin deeper exploration. 4. Animals acted to enhance creativity (play). 5. Companion animals increased the safety and comfort needed to investigate and experience the object world. 6. While playing with or stroking the pets, clients freely disclosed information regarding their past.	1. Stroking or receiving tactile comfort from an animal was observed to reduce anxiety, had a calming effect (noted being more relaxed). 2. Clients formed an attachment to therapy animal. 3. Animals seemed to provide a sense of safety and comfort in both children and adult clients. 4. Animals soothed clients and helped them remain calm while exploring difficult emotions. 5. Animals and clients displayed reciprocity in the nurturing that occurred; therefore, animals may have acted as a mature transitional object or transitional being. 6. Clients sought physical contact and displayed ritualistic behaviors such as rubbing, hugging, kissing, holding, and cuddling. 7. Clients displayed proximity-seeking, initiating interactions, expressing affection, and thinking about the object of attachment.

Chapter 6

SAVORING AND SHARING THE TREASURED FIND

IMPLICATIONS FOR THE PRACTICE OF COUNSELING AND PSYCHOLOGY

Enhancing the Therapeutic Relationship and Environment

This book supports the literature suggesting companion animals enhance the therapeutic relationship and therapeutic environment. The common denominator among all approaches used in counseling and psychology is the value placed on the client-therapist relationship (Corey, 2001). Researchers have indicated that approximately 30 percent of the variance in the therapeutic outcome of clients is directly affected by the therapeutic relationship (Gatson, 1990; Lambert, 1992; Najavitis & Strupp, 1994). Current research into animal-assisted therapy suggests that pets, especially dogs, enhance the therapeutic relationship through reduction of anxiety and arousal, acting as catalysts or mediators of human social interactions, providing nonjudgmental unconditional positive regard, and acting as outlets for nurturing behavior (Kruger & Serpell, 2006). With the client-therapist relationship being vital to the therapeutic process, it would seem a companion animals could, in some cases, be as one participant stated, "worth [their] weight in gold."

> ". . . anything that we can do to bring people in and enhance the working alliance are benefits to therapy. . . . anything we can do to reduce hopelessness . . . So why not have it if it's available . . ."

One of the difficulties with correlating research into the animal-human bond stems from a lack of theoretical conceptualizations (Brown, 2004). Questions arise as to "why" and "how" the human-pet bond is beneficial to clients during counseling and psychology. In applying the themes derived from the results of the project to Winnicott's object relations based concepts of the holding environment and transitional phenomena, the evidence suggested that the animals involved in therapy with the participants may have brought about positive changes in the therapeutic process by supplying elements inherent in the transitional phenomena of the good-enough-mother. It was found by acting as transitional beings or mature transitional objects, the animals provided the felt sense of safety needed for clients to work within the transitional space of the holding environment.

For Winnicott, and those who were influenced by his work, treatment was first and foremost "the provision of a congenial milieu" (Phillips, 1988, p. 11). The holding environment allows for the safety needed for clients to enter the transitional space where they can confront difficult issues and painful emotions in order to grow in self-awareness. The participants noticed that the animals used in therapy seemed to remove the barriers that were preventing clients from doing therapeutic work. The therapists noticed that clients were able to express and feel genuine emotions in relation to the issues causing them distress. Within Winnicott's view of the holding environment, the therapist or counselor takes on a sort of parental function. Perhaps the animals assisted the therapist through providing what appeared to be empathic mirroring and resonance, unconditional acceptance and love, warmth and comfort through affectionate touch and nurturing, and a sense of safety and protection, all of which represent qualities of the devoted good-enough-mother.

Participants stated that they had observed their animals acting as a bridge, linking them to detached, emotionally flat, defensive, and traumatized clients whom the therapists had been unable to reach. According to the participants, the animals seemed to be the key or the "smoking gun" with some clients when their attempts to develop a working alliance were unsuccessful. An example can be seen in this therapist's experience of having the dog link him to a client he had previously been unable to engage in therapy. After some time, he decided to try animal-assisted therapy and said, "*Then this dog came in. . . . That was my first sign of life. Wow!*" Could it be that the animals were able to, as stated by Melson and Fine (2006), "slip under the radar of human defense mechanisms" (p. 212)?

The cat and dogs in this project were observed to greet clients with enthusiasm, which was usually reciprocated with smiles and physical affection. Perhaps it was the animal's ability to make a client feel he or she was truly accepted, "warts and all." Companion animals often help humans release their judgments of themselves because they do not judge (Guerrero, 2003/2004). Without the fear of rejection, the clients could ease up on protecting themselves through their various defense mechanisms.

According to Fox (1981), many people find it easier to develop a relationship with an animal than with another human being. Human insecurities, ego defenses, and associated expectations and attitudes can be a barrier, and these are absent or at least minimal with a pet. Thus, facilitating the establishment of a natural, transpersonal relationship through a pet's unconditional openness and receptivity can lead to a "need-dependency relationship" satisfying such human needs as to mother, to be mothered, to indulge, or to dominate (p. 33). One could wonder if the animal's ability to connect the therapist with defensive or detached clients came from the pets satisfying the need of clients to feel "mothered," thus allowing for what was referred to by participants as a "breakthrough."

This book is not meant to suggest animal-assisted therapy is a panacea. However, as stated by Fine and Mio (2006), skilled therapists may use animal-assisted therapy as one of the tools at their disposal. They stated, "with the sensitive use of animals, they may very well achieve a therapeutic breakthrough" (p. 514). The evidence collected from the participants coincides with Fine and Mio's statement. Therapists spoke of breakthroughs that appeared to occur with certain clients when the animals were introduced into the treatment plan.

The Use of Animal-Assisted Therapy in Trauma

Participants provided evidence suggesting that the cat and dogs present in the therapy room were extremely helpful in providing the safety needed for traumatized clients to heal. One participant spoke of his experience working with a young woman who had experienced "extreme abuse" throughout her childhood. He stated, "*I would not have been able to do the therapy without the dog in the room.*" It was this psychologist's belief the "*dog was absolutely needed for things to be safe.*" From this participant's comment, one could conclude the animal acted to bring the safety needed to create a holding environment for this traumatized young woman.

The symptoms of traumatic stress disorders fall into three main categories. These are called hyperarousal, intrusion, and constriction (Herman, 1997, p. 35). In hyperarousal, the traumatized person startles easily, reacts irritably to small provocations, and sleeps poorly (p. 35). Clients can suffer from a combination of generalized anxiety symptoms and fears. The results presented in this book suggest the cat and dogs helped clients reduce anxiety by providing comfort and a sense of safety, often appearing to act as mature transitional objects or transitional beings, which act as agents of the good-enough-mother.

In states of hyperarousal, traumatized individuals can be highly sensitive to "slights" of any kind (Slochower, 1996). If the therapist triggers this sensitivity, a disruption in treatment can occur through the breakdown of safety inherent in the holding process. The evidence provided in this project suggests that the animals were able to maintain the holding environment when the psychologists could not. This makes one wonder whether the therapy animals would be able to act as a sort of backup for the therapist in the event that there is a break in the holding between client and therapist. The ability of the animals to maintain the connection with clients could be very significant in preventing the breakdown of holding with not only traumatized clients but also dependent and narcissistic clients who are also extremely sensitive to changes in the therapists' responsiveness (Slochower 1996).

The second symptom of trauma is intrusion. This causes an arrest in the course of normal development by its repetitive intrusion into the life of the survivor. The memories of the event lack verbal narrative and context, which makes processing the trauma difficult. The memories are, however, encoded in the form of vivid sensations and images stored in the limbic system and right hemisphere of the brain (Herman, 1997). In the treatment of trauma, creative therapy, such as art, is used to connect left brain cognitive abilities with the creative right brain, where the traumatic memory resides. The therapist can use the art project to assist clients to process the imagery and thus give voice to the memory. In doing so, the client can begin to integrate and heal from the traumatic injury (J. Simington, personal communication, 2006). The results suggest the participating cat and dogs brought an enhanced sense of safety, which appeared to enhance the clients' ability to be creative. This could be viewed as providing the opportunity to work within the transitional space.

Constriction is the third symptom of trauma. The survivor develops a detached state of consciousness that is similar to a hypnotic trance.

This leaves the person in a dissociative state where the perceptions of pain, and the normal emotional responses to pain, are severed (Herman, 1997). The participants observed detached clients come to life, engage, or open up when the animal was introduced into the treatment plan. They stated that the animals appeared to remove barriers walling off clients from their treatment.

> *"I could try and facilitate some sort of a dialogue that was genuine, but . . . response . . . very shallow . . . lack of any substance, genuineness. . . . Emotionally flat is also another aspect. . . . I think animal-assisted therapy has . . . been really, really working."*

In a state of dissociation a person can experience intense emotion yet not have clear memory of the event, or the person can remember everything in detail but without emotion. This fragmentation tears apart a complex system of self-protection that normally functions in an integrated fashion (Herman, 1997). Dissociation keeps traumatic memories out of ordinary consciousness, only allowing a fragment of the memory to emerge as an intrusive symptom. When dissociated, clients are "disconnected" and cannot do healing work (J. Simington, personal communication, 2006). The companion animals in this project were able to connect with detached and emotionally flat clients. Thus, it may be possible that the animals could help ground dissociated clients. Along with this, the animals appeared to provide an enhanced opportunity for creativity, which could be viewed as opportunities for trauma survivors to work in the transitional space where integration can occur.

Brown and Katcher (1997) found a positive correlation between companion animal attachment and dissociation. In their 2001 study, however, they also discovered that subjects with very high pet attachment scores were much more likely to have clinical levels of dissociation than did those subjects with lower pet attachment. (It is important to note that most participants in their study with high levels of pet attachment did not have clinical levels of dissociation.) According to Johnson, Odendaal, and Meadows (2002), this pet attachment occurs both with and without pet ownership.

Reviews of literature show that higher levels of dissociation are strongly correlated with previous traumatic experiences in both adults and children (Carlson, Armstrong, Loewenstein & Roth, 1998). Since dissociation correlates with pet attachment, Brown and Katcher (2001) believed it was possible that a subset of people highly attached to companion animals would have histories of abuse or trauma. With this in mind, it would seem probable that these individuals, who have high pet attachment or high levels of dissociation, could benefit a great deal by having a pet present during therapy sessions. Marguerite McCormack, who worked with the traumatized children involved in the 1999 Columbine High School tragedy, points to a very specific therapeutic benefit.

> Trauma does damage the ability to form a relationship. . . . It destroys the belief in a safe universe. If you don't have a sense of trust or a sense of safety, how can you form a relationship? Animals are safe. This is a relationship that will not bring you harm. In the fold of this relationship with the animal, it is possible to develop a vision of a life where you are calm, people are nice, and the universe is in its right place (McCormack, as cited in Becker, 2002, p. 51).

People who have been traumatized are in spiritual distress, and much of what is happening in the field of trauma recovery today focuses on spiritual connection (Staker, Watson & Robinson, 2002; Simington, 1996, 2003, 2005; Simington & Victorian Order of Nurses, 1999). Ordinary systems of care that provide people with a sense of control and meaning in their lives become overwhelmed when traumatic events occur. Ellison (1983) emphasized that it is the spirit of human beings that enables and motivates us to search for meaning and purpose in life and to seek what transcends us. Spirituality is described by Clark and Olson as "*an experience of being in relationship with*" (2000, p. 21). The detached trauma client is unable to connect in relationship to self, other, or the Creator, which results in difficulty with regard to meaning and purpose.

In spiritual distress, clients need the unconditional positive regard, genuineness, congruence, and empathy inherent in Taylor's (1991) concept of presence. They also need the unconditional positive regard and empathetic mirroring inherent in agape. In having someone witness their pain and bring hope through responding therapeutically to their suffering, clients can begin to heal (Ashbrook, 1996). In viewing this through Ashbrook's (1996) theological view of the holding environment, the evidence seemed to suggest the animals may have provided presence and agape. Nicoll (2005) has noticed that pets can provide a level of soul healing that cannot be obtained by the clinical examination of life events. Could it be the animals are able to supply a connection to spirit by creating a sacred transitional space within a warm and safe holding environment? An example of the animal's influence on the therapeutic milieu can be seen in the following statement of one of the participants,

> *"There is like a sense of peacefulness when the three of us are sitting in here. And it really helps too when there is that peacefulness and calm because then, when we have to tackle the tough issues — then we've already laid a foundation — you know it's okay to talk about these things."*

Companion Animals Enhancing the Work Environment

The participants provided evidence suggesting the companion animals enhanced their sense of well-being in the work environment. They believed the animal's presence made them appear friendlier and softer with clients, added to their productivity and creativity during the therapeutic encounter, and served to keep them grounded. From this description, one could conclude the animals may serve to decrease the incidence of burnout with these psychologists while enhancing positive therapeutic encounters.

SUGGESTIONS FOR FUTURE RESEARCH

One of the difficulties pertaining to research in the area of animal-assisted therapy is that the data bases of evidence do not have a key term or index term for human-animal interactions. The literature is widely dispersed making peer-reviewed research-quality publications difficult to unearth. Wood (2006) presents the techniques and strategies for searching for this information in a chapter in Fine's (2006) newly published *Handbook on Animal-Assisted Therapy* (2nd ed). This should prove helpful to those conducting future research in this area.

Five recommendations for future research surfaced as a result of this study. They will each be discussed as follows.

1. Animal-Assisted Therapy and the Holding Environment

This book was aimed at gaining an understanding into the possible roles a companion animal could play in therapy sessions with clients through the lens of Winnicott's concepts of the holding environment and transitional phenomena. This was done in an attempt to explain how companion animals may affect the therapeutic process, and what it is they may provide in the therapeutic setting.

In viewing the results of this project through the lens of philosophy, it would seem the findings were more akin to that of supplying metaphysical proof, rather than the empirical proof needed for an epistemological perspective. From a metaphysical perspective, researchers seek to develop a "knowing" in regard to the existence of proof (Fine & Mio, 2006, p. 518). However, in order to secure respectability as effective evidence-based intervention, it would seem a more acceptable research project would have to include empirical evidence.

Many involved in researching the effects of animals on clients in therapy believe qualitative studies are less causal research methods and are not in keeping with the current trend for evidence-based medicine (Wilson, 2006). The opinion of many researchers is that nonrandomized trials and observational studies are "more sophisticated;" while the gold standard is randomized controlled trials (Wilson, 2006, p. 504). Since the professional community is heading toward evidence-based practice (Eddy, 2005), Fine and Mio (2006) suggested that "a methodology needs to establish a track level of acceptable proof that supports its position" in order to secure respectability as an effective evidence-based intervention (p. 518).

Fine and Mio believed a small qualitative study such as this project "can point toward a trend and help researchers generate hypotheses to examine" (2006, p. 522). It is hoped that the qualitative description supplied in this book will plant a seed for future research into the effects of animal-assisted therapy on the holding environment and transitional phenomena. Larger qualitative studies could be conducted looking at the lived experience of both clients and therapists who have had companion animals present during therapy sessions. With the addition of questionnaires that address the companion animals' effects on transitional phenomena and the holding environment, statistical data could also be collected to provide the preferred proof needed for an epistemological perspective. This could aid in supplying the more evidence-based results of traditional quantitative studies.

2. Application to Other Theoretical Frameworks of Counselling and Psychology

It would be interesting to conduct studies focused on the role of companion animals within all individual theoretical frameworks of counseling and psychology. Practitioners could conduct small qualitative studies to illuminate aspects of animal-assisted therapy as they pertain to their choice of therapy base.

The Role of Companion Animals in Counseling and Psychology

Family systems theoretical frameworks could also be applied using therapy animals or having the companion animal dwell within the family unit. Fox (1981) noted that some of the behavioral problems that companion animals develop are linked with emotional troubles within the family or stem directly from the owner. He stated, "Family therapy involving the animal as well is now becoming a reality" (p. 35).

Although these small qualitative studies would not meet the gold standard of randomized controlled trials (Wilson, 2006), they could shed light on how animals could play a role within various theoretical frameworks. Qualitative research supplies the richness of coming to understand the lived experience of people. So much of life is mystery, and in becoming too focused on "scientific methods," we lose the gifts of the unexplainable. It seems Boris Levinson, a leader in researching the concept of animal-assisted psychotherapy, agreed. He stated,

> On the one hand, our science's feet touch problems that might well be investigated by rigorous, scientific experimentation, while, on the other hand, its head reaches into the clouds where measurement cannot bring answers and intuition must reign. After all, science brings us knowledge through the medium of our senses, and this is mighty little. If we forget how much we cannot "know" in this way, we become insensitive to many happenings of great importance in the relationship between man, animal, and the rest of nature. It seems to me, therefore, that in our seeking for new knowledge there are two distinct and yet related paths that we must follow. One is the so-called intuitive (the folk way) of studying the animal, the way used by the artist, poet, writer, plain people for generations; the other is so-called scientific. Both, in my opinion, are equally valid and equally worthwhile. The intuitive method looks at an animal as a teacher and friend; the scientific method looks at him as an object of curiosity. (1983, pp. 537–538)

3. Animal-Assisted Therapy and Trauma

Another suggestion for future research would be an investigation into the effects of companion animals on traumatized clients. Anecdotal reports have been written on the profound role therapy animals appeared to play in the aftermath of the "9-11" bombing of the Trade Centers in New York City (Kundera, 2005), the 1995 bombing of the Murrah Federal building in Oklahoma City (Chandler, 2006), the 1999 Columbine High School shootings, and the 1998 Thurston High School shooting in Springfield, Oregon (Becker, 2002). Survivors of trauma could be interviewed, polled, or provided with a questionnaire one to two years post the traumatic incident in order to gain understanding into what the companion animals supplied the victims and how that could be incorporated into future trauma treatment programs.

4. Matching Animals and Clients

Animal-assisted therapy has achieved considerable recognition among health professionals. However, animal-assisted therapy may not be suitable in all instances (McNicholas & Collis, 2006). Benefits arising from the contact with animals may be highly dependent on an individual's former or current pet ownership and level of ease felt in the company of animals. Not all individuals respond similarly. The attitudes a person holds toward an animal can have an impact on the stress-buffering effects of the presence of an animal. Studies have found that cardiovascular stress responses in the presence of a dog were significantly lower for people who thought of dogs more positively than they were for those with a more negative attitude (Freidmann & Tsai, 2006). New research should now be aimed at identifying those for whom programs involving pets would be successful and the mechanisms that underlie successful implementation.

For the purpose of the project contained in this book, companion animals, such as cats and dogs, were used because it would seem they are more anthropomorphically able to provide qualities of the good-enough-mother. However, many researchers have studied the effects of other species on humans, as well the effects of nature. Hunt, Hart and Gomulkiewicz (1992) reported an increase in social interactions when those who used parks brought a pet rabbit or a turtle with them. Studies on birds indicate they act as a social lubricant or ice breaker with elderly adults (Mugford & McComisky, 1975). Despite the high attrition rate in the study, the elderly adults who owned pet birds appeared to show social and psychological improvements as a result. Greer, Pustay, Zaun, and Coppens (2001) investigated the effect of cats on specific elements of communication and found an increase in all three communication measurements used.

Fish in tanks (Katcher, Segal & Beck, 1984), trees in parks (Ulrich 1984), and finches in a communal cage (Beck, Seraydarian & Hunter,

1986) have all been demonstrated to have effects on human health and well-being. However, research is needed to investigate which animals provide what benefits and which clients will benefit from what animals. This could provide the evidence needed to formulate a more individualized treatment plan for any given client.

5. Effects of Animal-Assisted Therapy on the Work Environment

Future research could be focused on the effects of the pets on therapists who use animal-assisted therapy in conjunction with their practice of counseling and/or psychology. This was a "surprise" discovery and could be further explored using empirical research methods such as monitoring physiological changes.

PROFESSIONAL AND ETHICAL CONSIDERATIONS

"Using any animal as part of [a treatment] plan needs to be done with appropriate care by studying the research on outcomes and keeping the safety of the client and animal in mind" (Parshall, 2003, p. 53). The goals of the client must be considered foremost. "The therapist must have the knowledge to assess the needs of the clients in relation to the therapeutic animal contact, to utilize the appropriate animal and/or activity and to evaluate the results of contact (Hoelscher & Garfat, 1993, p. 87). The counselor or psychologist incorporating an animal into his or her practice must be flexible. If the animal and client are not interacting beneficially, appropriate steps, such as removing the animal, need to be taken, and an alternate plan put into place.

The therapist must be aware of any fears, allergies or concerns, and provisions for an informed consent that must be made. In the event an animal becomes ill or dies, it is also important that the clinician has a plan devised for handling the explanation to children. There is also the potential risk of an animal injuring a client by biting or knocking them down. However, Parshall (2003) reports there are no reports in research articles or interviews indicating aggressive behavior on the part of either the animals used or the clients, residents, inmates, or patients involved in animal-assisted therapy programs. The participants involved in this project had never encountered any problems

Animal Welfare

Those using animal-assisted therapy have an ethical responsibility to ensure the safety and well-being of the animals that work as therapeutic adjuncts (Serpell, Coppinger & Fine, 2006). Animal-assisted therapy can be stressful to animals, perhaps for no other reason than the shift in their daily routine. Setting and schedule changes need to be monitored to ensure the animals are able to cope comfortably and are continuing to enjoy interactions with people. The therapist or handler must become adept at identifying behaviors that may indicate the animal is feeling distressed.

The clinician or handler must also remain aware of the animal's need for food, water, quiet time, and exercise during any given therapeutic day. If the animal shows signs of stress, it needs to be removed to a safe place. In the case of handler-dog teams, the handler can take the animal out of the room. If the animal belongs to the therapist, it is suggested a kennel be kept at work so the animal has its own safe "den" to hide away in and rest (Fredrickson-MacNamara & Butler, 2006).

Animal-assisted therapy is not appropriate if the emotional or activity levels of targeted populations are overwhelming to available animals. There is always a risk associated with exposure to potentially unpredictable clients. The animals need to be kept safe from any possibility of abuse or danger from clients at all times. As stated by McNicholas and Collis, "Any benefits to people that derive from animal contact require constant vigilance for the animal's well-being" (2006, p. 69). In the realm of individual and family therapies, animals used are usually the therapist's own pet, or the pet is accompanied by its handler/owner. Since either the therapist or handler owns the pet, responsibilities and obligations attending this type of animal-assisted therapy are comparable to those attending pet ownership.

Therapy pets need to be free from pain, injury, and disease. The animals should be up-to-date in their inoculations and have regular exams and supervision from a qualified veterinarian. A study done by Haubenhofer, Most, and Kirchengast (2005) has supplied valuable evidence toward ensuring the effects of therapy programs are not stressful to animals. They examined the levels of salivary cortisol in therapy dogs undergoing a five-day training course and found that the dogs did not experience stress during the performance of therapy-related tasks (as cited in McNicholas & Collis, 2006).

Wishon (1989) reported that most cats and dogs carry human pathogens, which have been associated with zoonotic diseases. However, Hines and Fredrickson (1998) point out that transmission has been extremely minimal. Many acute care hospitals in the United States have now incorporated animals into all areas of medical and surgical treatment with the exception of the actual operating room (Miller, 2000). "Animal-assisted therapy programs appear to cause few health problems for people, and most therapists feel that the programs are an acceptable risk if it lessens the despair that comes with loneliness" (Beck & Katcher, 1996, p. 130).

Animal Selection

Animals used in the field of animal-assisted therapy need to be well-trained and trustworthy. In Canada, one way to minimize the risk of inappropriate animal selection is to have the companion animals certified as Canine Good Citizens through the Canadian Kennel Association. Along with behavior testing, the animal should be checked by a veterinarian to assess the animal's physical well-being. Parshall (2003) believed the reason there have been no reports of aggressive behavior in therapy animals is because therapists and handlers have their animals certified by one of the relevant licensing agencies in any given country.

Not all animals are appropriate to work as therapy pets, just as not all humans make good therapists. Even the Dalai Lama reminded his readers that the degree of compassion held by dogs is just as variable as it is in humans (Dalai Lama, 2000). Therapy pets must be healthy, well-behaved, not aggressive toward people or other animals, friendly, and sociable and have a high tolerance for stress. Unsuitable, unhealthy, poorly behaved, nervous animals can be hazardous both physically and psychologically to an individual (Duncan, 1998; Edney, 1995). Each of the participants discussed the animals that are appropriate to use within the therapeutic setting. One therapist stated,

> *"there's a certain degree of unpredictability – and so I think we need to be careful about that. So it's really important that any animal that is chosen, we have a good sense of what their history is and what their predictability is."*

Client Selection

There is also a need to screen clients in order to assess whether they will benefit from animal-assisted therapy. It is necessary to obtain information about previous pet ownership and the attitudes held toward certain animals. In certain cases, such as clients with allergies related to the therapy animal, clients who have had bad experiences in the past with animals, and clients who do not like animals, the animals should not be used.

The animal's safety is of utmost importance. People with a history of animal abuse are not recommended for animal-assisted therapy programs. This is not only to protect the physical well-being of the animal but also for the animal's mental health. Animals are highly sensitive and intuitive. Thus, they may sense the client's abusiveness toward animals. An example can be seen through a situation that arose during an initial session of therapy with one of the therapists involved in the Chimo project. On entering the room, an experienced therapy dog began acting frightened in regard to a new male adolescent client. The handler removed the animal because he was showing signs of distress. This animal had never behaved in such a manner in the past, so the therapist did some investigating. It was discovered that the child had a long history of animal abuse. The parents had lied to the therapist on intake, thinking exposure to the dog might help their son to stop abusing other animals.

The participants in this study who worked with at-risk adolescents stated they were very particular in selecting clients. One psychologist stated,

> *"There needs to be a sense of trust between me and my client. If I think this client is unpredictable, if he has a history of abusing animals or is not going to conduct himself appropriately in session, then I would be very apprehensive . . . that comfort needs to be established before I select them for animal-assisted therapy."*

The three psychologists involved in this research project stated that they had never had a negative experience working with the pets in their practice. Some clients were found to respond more positively, but they have never had an incident in which a client did not want the animal present. When asked about clients with allergies, one of the participants had experienced one child who could not be around his

112   *The Role of Companion Animals in Counseling and Psychology*

dog. The therapists stated that clients with allergies "were not a big deal" in their respective practices.

CONCLUSIONS

Having been educated within the Catholic school system, I often heard about "God's grace." Yet my broken childhood made the concept of grace rather difficult to grasp. As I grew to adulthood, I came to understand the basic meaning of this word, yet failed to integrate it with any experience in my life. However, in the process of completing this book, I have come to understand the meaning of grace through a spiritual awakening that occurred in the context of my relationships with my pets. It was an effect I could have never anticipated. It seems this piece of writing held a message from a Higher Power – one I had been desperately searching for and needed.

I had struggled for years with a fundamental doubt preventing me from fully trusting in a God who left me feeling so alone and afraid as a child. In coming to understand that I was not abandoned, I have healed something deep within. Having been able to break through this spiritual impasse, my view of childhood has shifted from one of loneliness and fear to one of salvation through an amazing gift of animal grace. As McGraw (2001) has often stated, it is not so much what happens to us, but how we interpret the experience. It appears a spiritual opportunity lay at the center of my interest in animal-assisted counseling and psychology.

It seems the intellectual power of coming to understand the profound role my canine companions had in my growth and development pales in comparison to the emotional and spiritual effect it has had on me. In coming to understand the powerful healing effect of the various animals in my life, I have come to truly understand what is meant when authors have referred to animals as "embodiments of grace and blessing" (McElroy, 1996; Randour, 2000).

Glaser (1998) wrote a humorous book filled with his perceptions of the philosophical musings of his dog Calvin. He writes of Calvin's thoughts on evolution and divinity:

> Recently, a scientific report claimed "definitively" that we dogs are descended from wolves. Now I'm quite willing to believe that humans evolved from apes, because they act like apes much of the time (I've

Savoring and Sharing the Treasured Find 113

been outside a singles bar). But I refuse to believe that I evolved from such a wild creature as a wolf – I'm much too refined for that. Rather I believe that I and other dogs were created by God and are made in God's image. We are God's mirror reflection. That's why God spelled backwards spells dog. Isn't that one of the first things you English-speaking humans notice, the spelling thing? And who else but God loves as unconditionally as a dog? We don't care who you humans are or what you humans do, as long as you take some time to be with us, praise us, worship us, and do our bidding occasionally. Isn't that god-like? Even when you treat us badly or forget we're around, the minute you turn about and give us the attention we deserve, we lick your faces and give you comfort. Isn't that divine? (p. 23).

I believe the comfort of a dog's lick is divine and also that it often involves divine intervention. In my own case, my pets' soft and gentle tongues seemed to act as a form of therapeutic or healing touch, where by the loving energy of the Creator was passed on to me, bringing healing and the feeling I was connected to another being. I felt loved unconditionally and was provided with a much-needed sense of belonging. This enabled me to experience being part of something greater than myself. I was able to experience relationship and this relationship allowed me to remain connected to the world around me.

All humans have a desire, whether they are conscious of it or not, to be more connected to all of creation. This "yearning for wholeness" (Masson, 1997, p. 41) is part of the human condition, and animals help us to recapture the relationship we have with the "All" of creation (Wilber, 1998, p. 64). Because animals are about attunement, attachment, connection, and compassion, they are able to keep us involved in relationship (Nicoll, 2005).

The ways of animals and how they heal us are mysterious, but I agree with McElroy, who believes that, given the opportunity, animals can "reach into our painful, hurtful places and mend and soothe" (1996, p. 111). My lived experience, the literature I have read, and the stories of participants involved in this project seem to indicate that animals could be some of the most accomplished and accessible healers we may ever encounter. As Mark Twain remarked long ago, human beings have a lot to learn from the "Higher Animals" (as cited in Kowalski, 1999, p. 19).

APPENDICES

Appendix A

DEFINITION OF TERMS

Agape: Agape means "God-with-us" (Phil. 2:4–8) (as cited in Ashbrook, 1996, p. 14). In counseling, mutual give and take is bracketed "for the sake of putting ourselves at the disposal of the well-being of others apart from our own needs" (p. 14). Theologically, unconditional positive regard and empathic mirroring suggest agape, the Greek word for love.

Animal-Assisted Activity: "Animal-assisted activity provides opportunities for motivational, educational, recreational, and/or therapeutic benefits to enhance quality of life. Animal-assisted activity is delivered in a variety of environments by specially trained professional, paraprofessionals, and/or volunteers in association with animals that meet specific criteria" (Delta Society, 2004, p. 10). Key features include absence of specific treatment goal; volunteers and treatment providers are not required to take detailed notes; visit content is spontaneous.

Animal-Assisted Interventions: "Any therapeutic intervention that intentionally includes or incorporates animals as part of the therapeutic process or milieu" (Kruger et al., 2004, p. 4).

Animal-Assisted Therapy: Animal-assisted therapy is a goal-directed intervention in which an animal that meets specific criteria is an integral part of the treatment process. Animal-assisted therapy is directed and/or delivered by a health or human service professional with specialized expertise and within the scope of practice of his or her profession. Key features include specified goals and objectives for each individual and measured progress (Delta Society, 2004).

Anthropomorphizing: Irvine describes anthropomorphizing as "the full-on projection of human characteristics" on to animals (Irvine, 2004, 74–75). An example can be seen in the attribution of loyalty and protectiveness when an animal is actually expressing sexual and territorial instincts (Noonan, 1998). Rivas and Burghardt (2002) stated, "Anthropomorph-

117

ism is defined as the attribution of human properties to nonhuman entities. Such entities can be supernatural (gods) or animate or inanimate nature" (p. 9).

Biophilia: Wilson believed that a tendency to seek out natural settings and affiliate with animals and plants is written in our genetic program (Newby, 1999). He defined this trait as "the innate tendency to focus on life and life-like processes" (Beck & Katcher, 1996, p. 1).

Chimo Project: The Chimo Project of Edmonton, Alberta, is a research-based program, the goal of which is to identify various ways that animals could effectively be used in the treatment of mental illness. It also promotes the study of animal-assisted therapy and is researching ways to incorporate animal-assisted therapy into the curriculum of schools of psychiatry, psychology, and other training for professionals and hospitals (Urichuk & Anderson, 2003).

Companion Animal: Sarmicanic (2004) stated the current use of the term companion animal as an alternative to pet further emphasizes the difference between the humans' relationships with animals that have been domesticated for economic purposes and the animals we choose to take into our homes and our hearts. The term companion animal became a popular alternative to the word pet in the 1990s. According to Irvine, 'companion animals' remain 'other' than human but in a sense worth honoring, rather than one of inferiority" (2004, p. 58).

Delta Society: Dr. Michael McCulloch established the Delta Society in the United States of America in 1977, drawing its membership from many disciplines. It is now the leading professional organization conducting research on the effects of animals on human health (Bustad, 2001). It is also a leader in providing training in animal-assisted therapy and is the main organization for certifying therapy animals in the United States (Kruger et al., 2004). The mission of the Delta Society is to improve human health through service and therapy animals (Delta Society, 2005).

Domestication: Kretchmer and Fox (1975) defined domestication as "that point at which the care, feeding and, above all, the breeding of a species comes under the control of man" (Messent & Serpell, 1981, p. 6).

Ethology: "Ethology can be defined as the observation, often comparative study of animal and/or human behavior" (Turner, 2000, p. 449).

Good-Enough-Mother: The good-enough-mother is the most important presence in the field of Winnicott's transitional phenomena and can be defined as "a protectively hovering spirit who, always striving to adapt to her infant's needs, provides a holding environment in which the infant is contained. Her perceptions mirror the infant, who utilizes this mirroring to organize its own perceptions" (Kahane, 1993, pp. 278-279).

Appendix A 119

Holding Environment: The term holding environment has to do with psychologically framing, holding, and contextualizing clients in such a way that they feel validated, encouraged, and supported (Phillips, 1988). This allows the client to feel safe enough to risk exploration and discovery. To Winnicott (1965), the term holding environment referred to the infant's early relationship with the mother. He believed that a mother's nurturing relationship with the infant provided a psychological scaffolding, or holding environment, for the infant to develop internal psychic structures. According to Winnicott, this early holding environment is replicated in the therapeutic process through the client's relationship with the therapist. In therapy, the client's internalization of the therapeutic relationship serves as scaffolding for the client's development of psychological structure.

Life-World: Husserl introduced the concept of life-world (Carr, 1977). This term refers to the realm of original self-experience that we encounter in an everyday sense. "Investigation of the life-world — the way a person lives, creates, and relates in the world — precedes phenomenological reduction" (Moustakas, 1994, p. 48).

Lived Experience: This is the world as the person immediately experiences it pre-reflectively. According to Van Manen (2001), "reflection on lived experience is always recollective; it is reflection on experience that is already passed or lived through" (p. 10).

Object Relations Theory: Object relations theory holds that the infant's experience in relationship with the mother, or primary caregiver, is the main determinant of personality formation. The infant's need for attachment to the primary caregiver is believed to be the motivating factor in the development of the infantile self (Scharff & Scharff, 1995). According to this theory, humans are influenced the most by past and current relationships to other individuals as a main force for life. External objects are those we relate to externally. An internal object may be a piece of psychic structure that influences the way we react to criticism or may be a piece of psychic structure that influences the way we react to rejection. Each object has an affect that accompanies it (Cashdan, 1988).

Pet: The word pet is "generally applied to animals that are kept primarily for social or emotional reasons rather than for economic purposes" (Serpell & Paul, 1994, p. 129).

Presence: This refers to "the art of being with another in a state of loving listening" (Rousell, 1999, p.38). Pastoral theologian Charles W. Taylor (1991) defined presence as encompassing openness, unconditional positive regard, genuineness, congruence between experience and expression, and capacity for empathy (Ashbrook, 1996).

Shamanism: The word shaman is derived from the language of the Tungus peoples of Siberia, where anthropologists and ethnologists assume shamanism originated. Shaman has been defined as "one who knows" or "a wise one" because of the ability to shift conscious awareness beyond the physical. As well as the Native American shamans, there are individuals from other races and traditions who have a "fundamental ability to transcend time and space and to experience things that cannot ordinarily be perceived physically." (Meadows, 2003, p. 2). Shamans are known in anthropological circles as individuals having an unusual affinity with the spirits of animals and nature. Those with shamanic powers have a special, almost symbiotic relationship with one or more animal helping-spirits who mediate between people and their unconscious world (Serpell, 2000b).

Transitional Being: Unlike intimate transitional objects such as a stuffed toys or blankets, a transitional being moves and shows intentional behavior that is more like a person. Importantly, they can never contradict the attributes projected onto them with words (Katcher, 2000).

Transitional Object: The transitional object represents the warmth and comfort of the mother-child bond. When a mother or caregiver leaves an infant, the child can easily become upset by the disappearance of their primary caregiver. To compensate for the sense of loss, a child will imbue some object with the attributes of the mother (Phillips, 1988). The transitional object also supports the development of the self, because it is used to represent the first "not me" object. The use of transitional objects continues through our lives as we imbue objects with meaning and memories that are associated with other ideas, places, and people (Winnicott, 1953).

Transitional Relationship: "In a transitional relationship a child or an adult takes the attributes of a purely subjective object, a fantasy object, and projects them onto some real entity in the external world" (Katcher, 2000, p. 469). Play is the movement of attributes of fantasy objects from an internal space to real objects in external space.

Transitional Space: This term represents the intermediate area between internal and external reality. Winnicott believed it is an intensely personal space due to the fact its existence depends on each individual's early life experiences. If children can use this realm to initiate a relationship with the world, first through transitional objects, and later through play and shared playing, a rich cultural experience and enjoyment of true creativity will open up to them (Winnicott, 1971/2005).

Appendix B

INTERVIEW CHECKLIST

- [ ] Are the questions clear in my mind?
- [ ] Do I have an interview guide ready?
- [ ] How do I want to contact the participants (e.g. telephone, mail, in person)?
- [ ] How long will an interview take?
- [ ] What kind of interview setting is most appropriate?
- [ ] How much do I want to say in that first contact?
- [ ] What kind of anonymity can I guarantee?
- [ ] What times do I have available for interviews and for reflections afterwards?
- [ ] Do I want participants to prepare in some way, to think about the topic beforehand, or to bring some documentation?
- [ ] What if they decline?
- [ ] What kind of follow-up will I provide (e.g. will they read and approve of their "story" in the project, will they read the full report and comment?)

Appendix C

AGREEMENT TO BE INTERVIEWED

I, _____, do hereby consent to be interviewed for the purpose of academic research by Jane Wilkes in partial fulfillment of the requirements for the degree of Master of Arts in Pastoral Psychology & Counseling from St. Stephen's College, Edmonton, Alberta.

The objective of the research is to develop an understanding of the lived experience of therapists who use companion animals in their practice of psychotherapy. The research will provide the basis for a Master's Thesis. It is hoped that the research findings will be helpful in understanding the role of companion animals within the therapeutic process of counseling and psychology.

The results of each audiotaped interview will be transcribed by a "blind" reviewer committed to confidentiality, and analyzed by the researcher. You will be considered to be a participant and as such will be invited to make subsequent suggestions for changes to your personal "story" to ensure that it accurately reflects what you have shared during your interview through your narrative. As a participant in the project, you will be asked to comment on both the presentation of the information, and the researcher's analysis of the data.

Anonymity of the participants will be maintained through the use of pseudonyms in all written documentation. Participants will have the right to ask that parts of the interview be excluded if they wish.

The audiotape and transcribed notes will be stored in a locked filing cabinet separate from any identifying information for confidentiality and either returned to the participant or destroyed following completion of the study.

Appendix C 123

Transcripts will be kept for five years for possible future use in peer-reviewed journal submission.

It is understood that as a volunteer participant, I have the right to rescind this agreement and withdraw from this project at any time without any consequence to myself.

Participant's Signature   Researcher's Signature

_____   _____

Date_____

Appendix D

AGREEMENT TO BE AUDIOTAPED

I agree to allow Jane Wilkes to audiotape our interview for the purpose of academic research in partial fulfillment of the requirements for the degree of Master of Arts in Pastoral Psychology & Counseling from St. Stephen's College, Edmonton, Alberta.

I understand this material will only be used for the purposes of academic research,and that such material will be transcribed for use in a research project. Tapes will either be returned to the participant or destroyed following completion of the research project. Transcriptions will be stored and kept without identifiable information in a locked filing cabinet for five years and may be used in possible future peer-reviewed journal submission. After five years, the transcriptions will be destroyed.

Participant's Signature   Researcher's Signature

_____   _____

Date_____

Appendix E

PERSPECTIVES AND DEMOGRAPHICS

PART I

Central Research Question

What is the companion animals' role within the therapeutic process of counseling and psychology?

Interview Questions

What is your experience of having a companion animal present during sessions with clients?

What value, if any, has been derived from the presence of the companion animal?

PART II RESPONDENT'S PERSPECTIVE ON HER CAREER

1. How do you define animal-assisted therapy?

2. What motivated you to utilize pets in your practice?

3. How did you come to be involved in pet-facilitated/assisted therapy?

4. Have you received any formal training in animal-assisted therapy?

5. What concerns, if any, do you have in regards to pet-facilitated/assisted therapy?

6. How do you care for the animal's health and well-being during sessions?

7. Are there any instances when you do not use the companion animal?

8. What have you experienced as advantages and disadvantages within the work environment when a companion animal is present?

Part III Demographic Information

1. What animals do you use in your practice?

2. What age group do you usually work with in your practice?

3. What is your animal's training level/certification?

4. What theoretical framework shapes your practice?

Appendix F

TRANSCRIBER'S AGREEMENT OF CONFIDENTIALITY

I, _____, do hereby consent to transcribe interview tapes used for the purpose of academic research by Jane Wilkes in partial fulfillment of the requirements for the degree of Master of Arts in Pastoral Psychology & Counseling from St. Stephen's College, Edmonton, Alberta.

I agree to keep all interview tapes and contents of the tapes safe and secure while in my possession. I also agree to maintain confidentiality in regards to the content of the interview tapes.

Transcriber's Signature   Researcher's Signature

_____   _____

Date_____

Appendix G

AGREEMENT OF CONFIDENTIALITY FOR INDEPENDENT JUDGE

I, _____, acting as independent judge, do hereby consent to keep confidential all findings of research transcriptions used for the purpose of academic research by Jane Wilkes in partial fulfillment of the requirements for the degree of Master of Arts in Pastoral Psychology & Counseling from St. Stephen's College, Edmonton, Alberta.

I understand the objective of the research is to develop an understanding of the lived experience of therapists who use companion animals in their practice of psychotherapy. The research will provide the basis for a Master's Thesis. It is hoped that the research findings will be helpful in understanding the role of companion animals within the therapeutic process of counselling and psychology.

Confidentiality will be upheld in regards to the information shared during the research by myself and the researcher. Confidentiality of the interview material will be maintained through the use of pseudonyms in all written documentation.

Independent Judge's Signature   Researcher's Signature

_____   _____

Date_____

Appendix H

DELINEATING UNITS OF MEANING

So which is unfortunate. But that is the way it goes and we do what we can do. I think it's a brilliant addition to therapy. I recognize it as an adjunct therapy. I love how it fits in with CBT. I love being able to encourage kids to develop coping thought for the animal first and then for themselves. I love asking the question, "Well, what would [Lucky] say to that?" "What do you think [Lucky] would think if you did that?" "How would [Lucky] feel if you decided to AWOL?"	9-I think it's a brilliant addition to therapy. 9-recognize it as an adjunct therapy. 9-fits in with CBT 9-develop coping thought for the animal first and then for themselves. 9-I love asking the question, "Well, what would [Lucky] say to that?" What do you think [Lucky] would think if you did that?" "How would [Lucky] feel if you decided to AWOL?"
What is it you like about that?	
Because I think that it is far easier for kids to interact with [Lucky] initially than it is for them to interact with me, because pets of course are full of that unconditional positive regard. They love you even if you're having a bad day and they don't care if your hair is messy and they don't care if you're weeping on the couch. Of course you have empathy or you wouldn't be doing this. But I think it's far easier for them to be looking at [Lucky] and talk to you than it may be with me initially. I think that's definitely beneficial.	9-easier for kids to interact with [Lucky] initially than it is for them to interact with me 9-pets of course are full of that unconditional positive regard They love you even if you're having a bad day and they don't care if your hair is messy and they don't care if you're weeping on the couch. 9-you have empathy But I think it's far easier for them to be looking at [Lucky] and talk to you than it may be with me initially. I think that's definitely beneficial.
So it's like a bridge.	*9-So it's like a bridge. Yeah! Absolutely*
Yeah! Absolutely. That's a good way to look at it. And it just provides them the opportunity to – they might not be able to for example – role play with me what they're going to say to their father who may be dying of cancer or who's abandoning them, but they can sit and tell [Lucky] what they're going to say. So that's another – it's a flexible way to integrate therapeutic exercises. Very safe. He's comforting to them too.	9- they might not be able to role play with me what they're going to say but they can sit and tell [Lucky] what they're going to say. 9-flexible way to integrate therapeutic

Appendix I

CLUSTERING UNITS OF MEANING

Clusters of Meaning to Themes
☐ Tape A   ☐ Tape B   ☐ Tape C   Numbers = transcription page numbers

3. Affection
  3 Affection
  3 Attention
  6 Welcoming from animal
  6 Welcoming from animal
  7 Welcoming of animal
  12 Touch/Affection
  12 Touch/Affection
  12 Touch/Affection
  22 Animal shows affection
  38 Animals can show emotions and react in a way that a therapist cannot
  40 Animals can show emotion and react when therapist cannot due to ethics
  6 Love: boy was able to show love to the dog
  7 Affection: boy able to show affection
  12 Animal accepts affection
  15 Therapeutic tool: dogs provide affection that therapists cannot ethically
       provide
  15 Affection: able to provide much-needed affection
  20 Affection; dog was on top of her
  3 Affection: greets with special affection
  6 Affection: gives his paw
  6 Connection: connected with client through touch and affection
  9 Affection: giving and receiving affection is important role for the dog
  9 Meets needs for affection: dog not bound by ethical code

130

Appendix I 131

9 Affection: gives people a chance to show affection
9 Affection: military environment very utilitarian but dog allows permission for military men to show affection and have affection returned

<u>4. Animal Empathy/Compassion</u>
26 Animals show empathy
36 Animals can show level of empathy in client
24 Empathy/Compassion: dog reacts to child's pain by crawling up and lying beside
24 Empathy: It's like the dog is trying to absorb the energy of the hurting child
6 Compassion
6 Compassion/empathy: client crying and dog sat in front and gave her a paw to hold paws
6 Compassion: moves close to client if he senses sadness
5 Natural: dog gives natural empathetic responses

Appendix J

THEMES[*]

I. Enhanced Therapeutic Alliance/Relationship
Increased Disclosure/Depth of Work: 40
   Bridge/Rapport Building/Icebreaker: 24
   Catalyst for Therapeutic Work: 21
Increased Trust: 19
   Increased Compliance: 13
Facilitates Communication: 8
   Reduced Resistance: 8
     Emotional Indicator of Client: 5 (used in family therapy for this reason)
Attention Increased (children): 7
Teaching/Improved Positive Behavior/Social Skills: 27
Teaching/Enhanced Boundaries: 18
     Teaching/Improved Communication Skills: 7
     Teaching/Improved Coping Skills: 4
     Teaching Empathy: 20
Healing: 7
   Use with Trauma: 6
Enhanced Positive Outlook/Hope/Well-Being: 20
   Enhanced Self-Esteem: 9
Identification/Personalization (use with connecting to story of client): 7
Use with Children and/or Adolescents grieving lost pets: 3
Decreased Sadness: 2
Decreased Loneliness: 1
Decreased Withdrawal: 1

---

[*]Numbers depict units of meanings.

Appendix J   133

II. Enhanced Therapeutic Environment

Environment Enhanced
   Nurturing: 40
   Increased Safety: 35
   Warmth/Friendly/Comfortable/Safety: 27
   Intuition/Sensitivity: 25
   Relaxed/Calm: 13
   Animal's "Presence": 14
   Unconditional Positive Regard: 14
   Unconditional Love: 6
   Empathy/Compassion: 8
   Therapeutic/Healing/Enhanced: 6
   Mirroring: 4
Genuineness: 2
   Grounding: 2
   Protection: 1
Transitional Space: Play and Creativity
   Increased Play: 16
   Role-Play: 2
   Analogies: 2
Transitional Phenomena
   Appears in Trance with Clients: 1
   Imagination: 4
   Soothing object that is cuddled, loved, give warmth: Transitional Object:
   Comforting/Calming: 39
   Touch (cuddled): 34
   Soothing/Calming/Comfort (gives warmth): 25
   Affection (love): 24
   Attachment (bond with the animal): 23
   Anxiety Reduction: 15
   Decreased Fear: 1
Biophilia (nature-nurture): 10

III. Creating a Sense of Sacredness

Positive Acclimations: 51
Peaceful Environment: 9
Sacred Moments: 4
Powerful Experience: 3
Connects to Soul: 3
Connection to God: 2
Theology of Animals: 1

IV. Enhanced Professional Practice

Adjunct Therapy:

    Use with Cognitive Behavior Therapy, Interpersonal Therapy, Narrative, Person-Centered Therapeutic Tool

    Aid for Therapeutic Exercises/Therapeutic Activities with Animal: 10

    Animal as Co-therapist: 3

    Role-Modeling: 12

    Asset to Therapist: 28

    Positive Changes in Office Environment: 7 (Therapist C)

    Ethical Practice

        Professional Ethics: 16

        Animal Safety: 12

        Animal Selection/Certification: 35

        Client Selection: 25

    Therapeutic Activities with Animal: 10

    Negatives Rare to None: 3

Appendix K

FINAL THEMES[*]

I. Enhanced Therapeutic Alliance/Relationship
a. Trust
Increased Disclosure/Depth of Work: 40 Increased Trust: 19 = 59
Bridge/Rapport Building/Icebreaker: 24 Facilitates Communication: 8 = 32
Increased Compliance/Decreased Resistance: 21 Attention/Engagement
Increased: 7 = 28
b. Catalyst for Enhanced Healing 21 = 77
Healing: 7
Catalyst with Trauma: 6
Enhanced Positive Outlook/Hope/Well-Being: 20
Enhanced Self-Esteem: 9
Decreased Sadness: 2
Decreased Loneliness: 1
Decreased Withdrawal: 1
Identification/Personalization (connecting to story of client): 7
Use with Children and/or Adolescents Grieving Lost Pets: 3

II. Enhanced Therapeutic Environment
a. Warm friendly Safe Environment = 94
Therapeutic/Healing/Enhanced: 6
Increased Safety: 35
Warmth/Friendly/Comfortable/Safety: 27
Protection: 1
Relaxed/Calm: 13
Nature-Nurture: 10
Grounding: 2

---

[*]Numbers depict units of meanings.

b. Unconditional Acceptance = 59
Positive Regard: 14
Love: 6
Empathy: Intuition/Sensitivity: 25
Empathy/Compassion: 8
Mirroring: 4
Genuineness: 2
c. Nurturing 40 = 215
Caring Sense of Presence: 14
Comforting/Calming: 39
Soothing Object (warmth, comfort, calm): 25
Anxiety Reduction: 15
Decreased Fear: 1
Touch (cuddled): 34
Affection (love): 24
Attachment (bond with the animal): 23
d. Creativity = 25
Transitional Space
    Increased Play: 16
    Role-Play: 2
    Analogies: 2
Transitional Phenomena
    Appears in Trance with Clients: 1
    Imagination: 4

III. Enhanced Professional Practice = 118
a. Adjunct Therapy 32
Use in cognitive behavior therapy, Interpersonal Therapy, Narrative, Person-Centered: Aid for therapeutic exercises, "presence"
Therapeutic Activities with Animal (cognitive behavior therapy): 10
Teaching/Improved Positive Behavior/Social Skills: 27
Teaching/Enhanced Boundaries: 18
Teaching/Improved Communication Skills: 7
Teaching/Improved Coping Skills: 4
Teaching Empathy: 20
Emotional Indicator of Clients: 5
Role-Modeling: 12
Animal as Cotherapist: 3
b. Asset to Therapist's Well-Being 28 = 35
Positive Changes in Office Environment: 7 (Therapist C)
IV.   Creating a Sense of Sacredness = 76
Positive Acclimations: 51

Appendix K 137

Sacredness: 4
Peaceful Environment: 9
Sacred Moments: 4
Powerful Experience: 3
Connects to Soul: 3
Connection to God: 2
Theology of Animals: 1

BIBLIOGRAPHY

Ader, R. L., Cohen, N., & Felten, D. (1995). Psychoneuroimmunology: Interactions between the nervous system and the immune system. *The Lancet, 345*, 99–103.

Alger, J. M., and Alger, S. F. (2003). *Cat Culture: The Social World of a Cat Shelter.* Philadelphia: Temple University Press.

Allen, J. G. (1995). *Coping with Trauma: A Guide to Self-Understanding.* Washington, DC: American Psychiatric Press, Inc.

Allen, K., Blascovich, J. Tomaka, J., and Kelsey, R. (1991). Presence of human friends and pet dogs as moderators of autonomic responses to stress in women. *Journal of Personality and Social Psychology, 61*, 582–589.

Allen, L., and Burdon, R. (1982). The clinical significance of pets in a psychiatric community residence. *American Journal of Social Psychiatry, 6*, 722–728.

Anderson, W. P., Reid, C. M., and Jennings, G. L. (1992). Pet ownership and risk factors for cardiovascular disease. *Medical Journal of Australia, 157*, 298–301.

Andrews, T. (2003). *Animal Speak: The Spiritual and Magical Powers of Creatures Great and Small.* St. Paul, MN: Llewellyn Publications.

Arehart-Treichel, J. (1982). Pets: The health benefits. *Science News, 121*, 220–223.

Armstrong, E. A. (1973). *Saint Francis: Nature Mystic.* Berkeley, CA: University of California Press.

Ashbrook, J. B. (1996). *Minding the Soul: Pastoral Counseling as Remembering.* Minneapolis, MN: Fortress Press.

Ashworth, P. D., Giorgi, A., and de Koning (Eds.) (1986). *Qualitative Research in Psychology.* Pittsburgh: Duquesne University Press.

Bachman, S., and Bachman, C. (2003). Pet therapy: Healing recovery and love [Online]. Retrieved May 10, 2003 from *Pawprints and Purrs* Web Site. Available: http://www.sniksnak.com/therapy.html

Barker, S. B., and Dawson, K. S. (1998). The effects of animal-assisted therapy on anxiety ratings of hospitalized psychiatric patients. *Psychiatric Services, 49*, 797–801.

Barker, S. B., Kniseley, J. S., McCain, N. L., and Best, A. M. (2005). Measuring stress and immune response in healthcare professional following interaction with a therapy dog: A pilot study. *Psychological Reports, 96*, 713–729.

Beck, A., and Katcher, A. (1996). *Between Pets and People: The Importance of Animal Companionship.* West Lafayette, IN: Purdue University Press.

Beck, A. M., and Katcher, A. H. (2003). Future directions in human-animals bond research. *American Behavioral Scientist, 47*, 79–93.

Beck, A. M., Seraydarian, L., and Hunter, G. F. (1986). The use of animals in the rehabilitation of psychiatric inpatients. *Psychological Reports, 8*, 63–66.

Becker, M. (2002). *The Healing Power of Pets: Harnessing the Amazing Ability of Pets to Make and Keep People Happy and Healthy.* New York: Hyperion.

Bekoff, M. (2001). The evolution of animal play, emotions and social mortality: On science, theology, spirituality, personhood, and love. *Zygon, 36*, 615–655.

Berl, M. E. (1952). Therapy at the zoo. *Quarterly Journal of Child Behavior, 4*, 209–212.

Birch, C., and Vischer, L. (1997). *Living with the animals: The community of God's creatures.* Geneva, Switzerland: WCC Publications.

Blue, G. F. (1986). The value of pets in children's lives. *Childhood Education, 24*, 85–89.

Boone, J. A. (1954/1976). *Kinship with all Life.* New York: HaprerCollins Publishers.

Borowski, O. (1998). *Every Living Thing: Daily Use of Animals in Ancient Israel.* Walnut Creek, CA: AltaMira Press.

Bossard, J. (1944). The mental hygiene of owning a dog. *Mental Hygiene, 28*, 408–413.

Bowlby, J. (1973). *Attachment and Loss: Vol 3. Sadness and Depression.* New York: Basic books.

Bowlby, J. (1988). *A secure base, parent-child attachment and healthy human development.* New York: Basic books.

Bowlby, J. (1989). *Secure and Insecure Attachment.* New York: Basic Books.

Brickel, C. M. (1979). The therapeutic roles of cats mascots with a hospital-based geriatric population. *The Gerontologist, 19*, 368–372.

Brickel, C. M. (1984). Depression in the nursing rooms: A pilot study using pet facilitated therapy. In R. R. Anderson and L. A. Hart (Eds.), *The Pet Connection* (pp. 407–415). Minneapolis: University of Minnesota Press.

Bridger, H. (May, 1970). *Companionship with Humans.* Paper presented to the Health Congress of the Royal Society of Health, Brighton.

Brown, B. H., Richards, H. C., and Wilson, C. A. (1996, May/June). Pet bonding and pet bereavement among adolescents. *Journal of Counseling and Development, 74*, 505–509.

Brown, J. P., and Silverman, J. D. (1999). The current and future market for veterinarians and veterinary medical services in the United States. *Journal of the American Veterinary Medical Association, 215*, 161–183.

Brown, S. (2004). The human-animal bond and self-psychology: Toward a new understanding. *Society & Animal, 12*, 67–86.

Brown, S., and Katcher, A. H. (1997). The contribution of attachment to pets and attachment to nature to dissociation and absorption. *Dissociation, 10*, 125–129.

Brown, S., and Katcher, A. H. (2001). Pet attachment and dissociation. *Society & Animals, 9*, 25–41.

Buber, M. (1996). *The Way of Response: Selections of His Writings.* (N. N. Glatzer, Ed.). New York: Schocken Books.

Buckley, P. (Ed.). (1986). Supportive psychotherapy. *Psychiatric Annals, 16*, 515–521.

Bustad, L. (1980). *Animals, Aging, and the Aged.* Minneapolis, MN: University of Minnesota Press.

Bibliography

Bustad, L. (1981). *Companion Animals and the Aged.* Symposium conducted at the International Conference on the Human-Companion Animal Bond, Philadelphia, PA.

Bustad, L. K. (2001).The importance of animals to the well-being of people. In P. Salotto (Ed.), *Pet Assisted Therapy: A Loving Intervention and an Emerging Profession: Leading to a Friendlier, Healthier and More Peaceful World* (pp. 272–277). Norton, MA: D. J. Publications.

Bustad, L. K., and Hines, L. M. (1982). Placement of animals with the elderly: Benefits and strategies. *California Veterinarian, 36,* 37–44.

Butler, K. (2004). *Therapy Dogs Today: Their Gifts, Our Obligation.* Norman, OK: Funpuddle Publishing Associates.

Carkuff, R. R. (1969). *Helping and Human Relations.* Amherst, MA: Human Resources Development Press.

Carlson, E. B., Armstrong, J., Loewenstein, R., and Roth, D. (1998). Relationships between traumatic experiences and symptoms of posttraumatic stress, dissociation and amnesia. In J. D. Bremner and C. R. Marmar (Eds.), *Trauma, Memory and Dissociation* (pp. 205–227). Washington, DC.: American Psychiatric Press.

Carmack, B. (Ed.) (1991). Introduction. *Holistic Nursing Practice, 5,* 1–2.

Carr, D. (1977) Husserl's problematic concept of the life-world. In F. Elliston and P. McCormick (Eds.) *Husserl expositions and appraisals* (pp. 202–212). Notre Dame, IN. University of Notre Dame Press.

Cashdan, S. (1988). *Object Relations Theory: Using the Relationship.* Markham, Ontario: Penguin Books (Canada).

Chandler, C. K. (2006). "Pawsitive" Pets: Working with Your Pet as Cotherapist (article 26) [Online]. Retrieved December 22, 2006 from Counseling Outfitters web site. Available: http://counselling outfitters.com/vistas/vistas06/vistas06.26.pdf

Chimo Project Final Team Report (2003, November). Retrieved February 2006 from *Angelfire* web site. Available: http://www.angelfire.com/mh/chimo/pdf/Final_Project_Team_Report-oct03.pdf

Clark, M. B., and Olson, J. K. (2000). *Nursing Within a Faith Community: Promoting Health in Times of Transition.* Thousand Oaks, CA: Sage Publications, Inc.

Coren, S. (2002). *The Pawprints of History: Dogs and the Course of Human Events.* New York, NY: Free Press.

Corey, G. (2001). *The Art of Integrative Counseling.* Belmont, CA: Thomson Brooks/Cole.

Corson, S., and Corson, E. (1977, January–February). Pet dogs as nonverbal communication links in hospital psychiatry. *Comprehensive Psychiatry, 18,* 61–72.

Corson, S., and Corson, E. (1978). Pets as mediators of therapy. *Current Psychiatric Theories, 18,* 195–205.

Corson, S., and Corson, E. (1980). Pet animals as nonverbal communication mediators in psychotherapy in institutional settings. In S. Corson and E. Corson (Eds.), *Ethology and Nonverbal Communication in Mental Health* (pp. 83–110). Oxford: Pergamon Press.

Corson, S. A., Corson, E. O., Gwynne, P. H., and Arnold, L. E. (1977). Pet dogs as

142 *The Role of Companion Animals in Counseling and Psychology*

nonverbal communication links in hospital psychiatry. *Comprehensive Psychiatry, 18*, 61–72.

Crawford, J. J., and Pomerinke, K. A. (2003). *Therapy Pets: Healing Partnership.* Amherst, NY: Prometheus Books.

Creswell, J. W. (1998). *Qualitative Inquiry and Research Design: Choosing Among Five Traditions.* Thousand Oaks, CA: Sage Publications.

Cusack, O. (1988). *Pets and Mental Health.* New York, NY: Haworth Press.

Dalai Lama (2000). *Ancient Wisdom, Modern World: Ethics for the New Millennium.* New York: Penguin Putnam.

Davis, J. H. (1987). Preadolescent self-concept development and pet ownership. *Anthrozoos, 1*, 90–94.

Davis, J. H., and Juhasz, A. M. (1995). The preadolescent/pet friendship bond. *Anthrozoos, 8*, 78–82.

Davis, S. J. M., and Valla, F. R. (1978). Evidence for domestication of the dog 12,000 years ago in the Natufian of Israel. *Nature, 276*, 608–610.

Delafield, G. (1975). *Self Perception and the Effects of Mobility Training.* Unpublished doctoral dissertation, University of Nottingham, United Kingdom.

Delta Society (2004). *Team Training Course Manual: A Delta Society Program for Animal-Assisted Activities and Therapy* (6th ed.). Bellevue, WA: Delta Society.

Delta Society (2005). Mission statement [Online]. Retrieved October, 2006. Available: http://www.deltasociety.org

DeMello, L. R. (1999). The effect of the presence of a companion-animal on physiological changes following the termination of cognitive stressors. *Psychology and Health, 14*, 859–868.

Dresser, N. (2000). The horse *bar-mitzvah*: A celebratory exploration of the human animal bond. In A. L. Podberscek, E. S. Paul, and J. A. Serpell (Eds.). *Companion Animals & Us: Exploring the Relationships Between People and Pets* (pp. 90–107). New York: Cambridge University Press.

Duncan, (1998). The importance of training standards for service animals. In C. C. Wilson and D. C. Turner (Eds.), *Companion Animals in Human Health* (pp. 251–266). Thousand Oaks, CA: Sage Publications.

Eaton, J. (1995). *The Circle of Creation: Animals in the Light of the Bible.* London, England: SCM Press Ltd.

Eddy, D. M. (2005). Evidence-based medicine: A unified approach. *Health Affairs, 24*, 9-17.

Eddy, J., Hart, L. A., and Boltz, R. P. (1988). The effects of service dogs on social acknowledgement of people in wheelchairs. *Journal of Psychology, 122*, 39–45.

Edenburg, N., and Baarda, B. (1995). The role of pets in enhancing human well-being: Effects on child development [Online]. In I. H. Robinson (Eds.), *Waltham Book of Human-Animal Interactions: Benefits and Responsibilities of Pet Ownership* (pp. 7-17). Retrieved May 10, 2003 from the Delta Society web site: Available: http://www.delta society.org/dsx211.htm

Edney, A. T. (1995). Companion animals and human health: An overview. *Journal of the Royal Society of Medicine, 88*, 704–708.

Eisner, E. W. (1991). *The Enlightened Eye: Qualitative Inquiry and the Enhancement of Educational Practice.* New York: Macmillan.

Bibliography 143

Ellison, C. W. (1983). Spiritual well-being: Conceptualization and measurement. *Journal of Psychology and Theology, 11,* 330–340.

Eriksen, W. (1994). The role of social support in the pathogenesis of coronary heart disease: A literature review. *Family Practice, 11,* 201–209.

Filiatre. J. C., Millot, J. L., and Montagner, H. (1983). New finding on communication behaviour between the young child and his pet dog. In *The Human Pet Relationship.* International Symposium on the Occasion of the 80th Birthday of Nobel Prize Winner Prof. Dr. Konrad Lorenz (pp. 50–57). Vienna: IEMT.

Farber, M. (1943). *The Foundation of Phenomenology.* Albany NY: SUNY Press.

Fine, A. (2000). Animals and therapists: Incorporating animals in outpatient psychotherapy. In A. H. Fine (Ed.), *Handbook on Animal-Assisted Therapy: Theoretical Foundations and Guidelines for Practice* (pp. 179–211). San Diego, California: Academic Press.

Fine, A. H. (Ed.) (2006). *Handbook on Animal-Assisted Therapy: Theoretical Foundations and Guidelines for Practice* (2nd ed.). San Diego, CA: Academic Press.

Fine, A. H., and Mio, J. S. (2006). The future of research, education, and clinical practice in the animal-human bond and animal-assisted therapy. Part C: The role of animal-assisted therapy in clinical practice: The importance of demonstrating empirically orientated psychotherapies. In A. H. Fine (Ed.), *Handbook on Animal-Assisted Therapy: Theoretical Foundations and Guidelines for Practice* (2nd ed.) (pp. 513–523). San Diego, CA: Academic Press.

Fogle, B. (1981). Attachment-euthanasia-grieving. In B. Fogle (Ed.), *Interrelations Between People and Pets* (pp. 331–342). Springfield, IL: Charles C Thomas. (In literature, Chief Seattle (c.1786–1866) may also be referred to by his Catholic baptismal name, Noah Sealth.)

Fox, M. (1981). Relationships between the human and nonhuman animals. In B. Fogle (Ed.), *Interrelations Between People and Pets* (pp. 23–40). Springfield, IL: Charles C Thomas.

Fredrickson-MacNamara, M., and Butler, K. (2006). The art of animal selection for animal-assisted activity and therapy programs. In A.H. Fine (Ed.), *Handbook on Animal-Assisted Therapy: Theoretical Foundations and Guidelines for Practice* (2nd ed.), (pp. 121–147). San Diego, CA: Academic Press.

Freud, S. (1952). *Totem and taboo: Some Points of Agreement Between the Mental Lives of Savages and Neurotics.* New York: W.W. Norton & Company.

Friedmann, E., Katcher, A. H., Lynch, J. J., and Thomas, S. A. (1980). Animal companions and one year survival of patients after discharge from a coronary care unit. *Public Health Reports, 95,* 307–312.

Friedmann, E., and Thomas, S. A. (1995). Pet ownership, social support, and one-year survival after acute myocardial infarction the Cardiac Arrhythmia Suppression Trial (CAST). *American Journal of Cardiology, 76,* 1213–1217.

Friedmann, E., and Tsai, C. (2006). The animal-human bond: Health and wellness. In A. H. Fine (Ed.) *Handbook on Animal-Assisted Therapy: Theoretical Foundations and Guidelines for Practice* (2nd ed.), (pp. 95–117). San Diego, CA: Academic press.

Furman, W. (1989). The development of children's social networks. In D. Belle (Ed.), *Children's Social Networks and Social Supports* (pp. 151-172). New York: John Wiley & Sons New York.

Gatson, L. (1990). The concept of the alliance and its role in psychotherapy: Theoretical and empirical consideration. *Psychotherapy, 27,* 143–153.

Gilbert, P. (1989). *Human Nature and Suffering.* Hillsdale, N.J.: Lawrence Erlbaum Associates.

Glaser, C. (1998). *Unleashed: The Wit and Wisdom of Calvin the Dog.* Louisville, Kentucky: Westminster John Knox Press.

Goldstein, M. (1999). *The Nature of Animal Healing: The Definitive Holistic Medicine Guide to Caring for Your Dog and Cat.* New York: Ballantine Books.

Greene, M. (1997). The lived world, literature, and education. In D. Vandenberg (Ed.), *Phenomenology & Educational Discourse* (pp. 169–190). Johannesburg: Heinemann.

Greer, K., Pustay, K., Zaun, T., and Coppens, P. (2001). A comparison of the effects of toys versus live animals on the communication of patients with dementia of the Alzheimer's type. *Clinical Gerontologist, 24,* 157–182.

Groenewald, T. (2004). A phenomenological research design illustrated [Online]. *International Journal of Qualitative Methods, 3,* 1–26. Article 4. Retrieved January 31, 2005 from the University of Alberta web site. Available: http://www.ulaberta.ca/~iiqm/back issues/3_1/pdf/groenewald.pdf

Guerrero, D. L. (2003/2004). *What animals can teach us about spirituality: Inspiring lessons from wild and tame creatures.* Woodstock, VT: SkyLight Paths Publishing.

Guttman, G., Predovic, M., AND Zemanek, M. (1983). The influence of pet ownership on non-verbal communication and social competence in children. In *The Human Pet Relationship.* International symposium on the occasion of the 80th birthday of Nobel Prize Winner Prof. Dr. Konrad Lorenz (pp. 58–63). Vienna: IEMT.

Harlow, H. F. (1959). Love in infant monkeys. *Scientific American, 200,* 68–74

Harper, T. (1994). *The Uncommon Touch.* Toronto: McClelland & Stewart.

Hart, L. A., Hart, B. L., and Bergin, B. (1987). Socializing effects of service dogs for people with disabilities. *Anthrozoos, 1,* 41–45.

Haubenhofer, D., Mostl, E., and Kirchengast S. (2005). Cortisol concentrations in saliva of humans and their dogs during intensive training courses in animal assisted therapy. *Wiener Tierarztliche Monatsschrift, 92,* 66–73.

Heiman, M. (1965). Psychoanalytic observation on the relationship of pet and man. *Veterinary Medicine/Small Animal Clinician, 60,* 713–718.

Heiman, M. (1967). The relationship between man and dog. *Psychoanalytic Quarterly, 25,* 568–585.

Herman, J. L. (1997). *Trauma and Recovery: The Aftermath of Violence—from Domestic Abuse to Political Terror.* New York, NY: BasicBooks.

Hines, L., and Fredrickson, M. (1998). Perspectives on animal-assisted activities and therapy. In C. C.Wilson and D. C. Turner (Eds.), *Companion Animals in Human Health* (pp. 23–29). Thousand Oaks, CA: Sage Publications, Inc.

Hines, L. M. (2003, September). Historical perspectives on the human-animal bond. *American Behavioral Scientist, 47,* 7–15.

Hoelscher, K., and Garfat, T. (1993). Talking to the animals. *Journal of Child and Youth Care, 8,* 87–92.

Bibliography

Holloway, I. (1997). *Basic Concepts for Qualitative Research.* Oxford: Blackwell Science.

Hooker, S. D., Freeman, L. H., and Stewart, P. (2002). Pet therapy research: A historical review. *Holistic Nursing Practice, 17,* 17–23.

Hunt, S. J., Hart, L. A., and Gomulkiewicz, R. (1992). Role of small animals in social interactions between strangers. *Journal of Social Psychology, 132,* 245–256.

Hycner, R. (1985). Some guidelines for the phenomenological analysis of interview data. *Journal of Human Studies, 8,* 279–303.

International Bible Society. (1984). *Holy Bible: New International Version.* Grand Rapids, MI: Zondervan Publishing House.

Irvine, L. (2004). *If You Tame Me: Understanding Our Connection with Animals.* Philadelphia: Temple University Press.

Jalongo, M. R. (2004). On behalf of children: From salamanders to Shetland ponies: Companion animals and young children. *Early Childhood Education Journal, 31,* 223–225.

Joachin, M. (2001). Future directions in pet assisted therapy: A drug prevention model. In P. Salotto (Ed.), *Pet Assisted Therapy: A Loving Intervention and an Emerging Profession: Leading to a Friendlier, Healthier, and More Peaceful World* (pp. 291–294). Norton, MA: D. J. Publications.

Johnson, R. A., Odendaal, J. S. J., and Meadows, R. L. (2002). Animal-assisted intervention and research: Issues and answers. *Western Journal of Nursing Research, 24,* 422–440.

Jones, B. (1985). *The Psychology of Companion Animal Bond: Animal Biographies.* Philadelphia: University of Pennsylvania.

Kahane, C. (1993). Gender and voice in transitional phenomena. In P. L. Rudnytsky (Ed.), *Transitional Objects and Potential Spaces: Literary Uses of D. W. Winnicott* (pp. 278–291). New York: Columbia University Press.

Kalsched, D. (2005). *The Inner World of Trauma: Archetypal Defenses of the Personal Spirit.* New York: Routledge.

Katcher, A. H. (1981). Interactions between people and their pets: Form and function. In B. Fogle (Ed.), *Interrelations Between People and Pets* (pp. 41–67). Springfield, IL: Charles C Thomas.

Katcher, A. H. (2000). Animal-assisted therapy and the study of human-animal relationships: Discipline or bondage? Context or transitional object? In A. Fine (Ed.), *Handbook on Animal-Assisted Therapy: Theoretical Foundations and Guidelines for Practice* (pp. 461–473). San Diego, CA: Academic Press.

Katcher, A. H., and Friedmann, E. (1980). Potential health value of pet ownership. In *Compendium on Continuing Education for the Veterinarian* (Vol. 2, pp. 117–121).

Katcher, A. H., Segal, H., and Beck, A. M. (1984). Comparison of contemplation and hypnosis for the reduction of anxiety and discomfort during dental surgery. *American Journal of Clinical Hypnosis, 27,* 14–21.

Kellert, S. R., and Wilson, E. O. (1993). The Biophilia Hypothesis. Washington, DC: Island Press.

Kidd, A. H., and Kidd, R. M. (1985). Children's attitudes toward their pets. *Psychological Reports, 57,* 15–31.

Kidd, A. H., and Kidd, R. M. (1990). Factors in children's attitudes toward pets. *Psychological Reports, 65,* 903–910.

Kirby. S., and McKenna, K. (1989). *Experience, Research, Social Change: Methods from the Margins.* Toronto: Garamond Press.

Knapp, C. (1998). *Pack of Two: The Intricate Bond Between People and Dogs.* New York: The Dial Press.

Kowalski, G. (1999). *The Souls of Animals* (2nd ed.). Walpole NH: Stillpoint Publishing.

Kretchmer, K. R., and Fox, M. W. (1975). Effects of domestication on animal behaviour. *Vet Rec, 96,* 102–108.

Kruger, D. (1988). *An Introduction to Phenomenological Psychology* (2nd ed.). Cape Town, South Africa: Juta.

Kruger, K. A., and Serpell, J. A. (2006). Animal-assisted interventions in mental health: Definitions and theoretical foundations. In A. H. Fine (Ed.) *Handbook on Animal-Assisted Therapy: Theoretical Foundations and Guidelines for Practice* (2nd ed.), (pp. 21–38). San Diego, CA: Academic press.

Kruger, K. A., Trachtenberg, S. W., and Serpell, J. A. (2004). Can animals help humans heal? Animal-assisted interventions in adolescent mental health [Online]. Retrieved July 4, 2005 from *The Center for the Interaction of Animals and Society University of Pennsylvania School of Veterinary Medicine web site.* Available: http://www2.vet.upenn.edu/research/centers/cias/pdf/CIAS_AAI_white_paper.pdf

Kundera, M. (2005). Willow and Rosie: The ordinary miracle of pets. In J. Canfield, M. V. Hansen, M. Becker, C. Kline, and A. D. Shojai (Eds.), *Chicken Soup for the Dog Lovers Soul.* Deerfield Beach, FL: Health Communications Inc.

Kvale, S. (1996). *Interviews: An Introduction to Qualitative Research Interviewing.* Thousand Oaks, CA: Sage.

Lambert, M. J. (1992). Implications of outcome research for psychotherapy integration. In J. C. Norcross and M. R. Goldstein (Eds.), *Handbook of Psychotherapy Integration* (pp. 94–129). New York: Basic Books.

Lasher, M. (1996). *And the Animals Will Teach You: Discovering Ourselves Through our Relationships With Animals.* New York: The Burkley Publishing Group.

Lawrence, B. (1967). Early domestic dogs. *Z Saugetierkd, 32,* 44–59.

Lawrence, E. (1993). The sacred bee, the filthy pig, and the bat out of hell: Animal symbolism as cognitive biophilia. In S. R. Kellert and E. O. Wilson (Eds.), *The Biophilia Hypothesis.* Washington, DC: Shearwater Press.

Levinson, B. (1962). The dog as a co-therapist. *Mental Hygiene, 46,* 59–65.

Levinson, B. (1964). Pets: A special technique in child psychotherapy. *Mental Hygiene, 48,* 243–248.

Levinson, B. (1965a). The veterinarian and mental hygiene. *Mental Hygiene, 49,* 3320–3323.

Levinson, B. (1965b). Pet psychotherapy: Use of household pets in the treatment of behavior disorder in childhood. *Psychological Reports, 17,* 695–698.

Levinson, B. (1969). *Pet-oriented Child Psychotherapy.* Springfield, ILL: Charles C Thomas.

Levinson, B. (1971). Household pets in training schools serving delinquent children. *Psychological Reports, 28,* 475–481.

Levinson, B. M. (1972). *Pets and Human Development.* Springfield, IL: Charles C Thomas Publisher, Ltd.

Levinson, B. M. (1975). Forecast for the year 2000. In R. S. Anderson (Ed.), *Pet Animals and Society* (pp. 155–159). London: Bailliere, Tindall.

Levinson, B. M. (1983). In A. Katcher and A. Beck (Eds.), *New Perspective on Our Lives With Companion Animals* (pp. 536–550). Philadelphia: University of Pennsylvania Press.

Levinson, B. M., and Mallon, G. P. (1997). *Pet-Oriented Child Psychotherapy* (2nd ed.). Springfield, IL: Charles C Thomas.

Loar, L., and Colman, L. (2004). *Teaching Empathy: Animal-Assisted Therapy Programs for Children and Families Exposed to Violence.* Alameda, CA: Latham Foundation Publication.

Lorenz, K. Z. (1952). *King Soloman's Ring.* London: Methuen.

Mader, B., Hart, L. A., and Bergin, B. (1989). Social acknowledgements for children with disabilities: Effects of service dogs. *Child Development, 60,* 1529–1534.

Mason, M. S., and Hagan, C. B. (1999). Pet-assisted psychotherapy. *Psychological Reports, 84,* 1235–1245.

Masson, J. (1997). *Dogs Never Lie About Love.* New York: Crown Publishers.

Maypole, J., and Davies, T. G. (2001). Students' perceptions of constructivist learning in a community college American History II. *Community College Review, 29,* 54–80.

McCulloch, M. J. (1981). The pet as prosthesis: Defining criteria for the adjunctive use of companion animals in the treatment of medically ill, depressed outpatients. In B. Fogle (Ed.), *Interrelations Between People and Pets* (pp. 101–123). Springfield, IL: Charles C Thomas.

McElroy, S. C. (1996). *Animals as Teachers and Healers: True Stories and Reflections.* New York: Random House.

McGraw, P. (2001). *Self Matters: Creating Your Life from the Inside Out.* New York: Simon & Schuster.

McNicholas, J., and Collis, G. M. (1998). Could Type A (coronary prone) personality explain the association between pet ownership and health? In C. C. Wilson and D. C. Turner (Eds.), *Companion Animals in Human Health* (pp. 173–186). Philadelphia: University of Philadelphia Press.

McNicholas, J., & Collis, G. M. (2000). Dogs as catalysts for social interactions: Robustness of the effect. *British Journal of Psychology, 91,* 61–70.

McNicholas, J., and Collis, G. M. (2006). Animals as social supports. In A. H. Fine (Ed.), *Handbook on Animal-Assisted Therapy: Theoretical Foundations and Guidelines for Practice* (2nd ed.) (pp. 49–71). San Diego, CA: Academic Press.

Meadows, K. (2003). *Shamanic Experience: A Practical Guide to Psychic Powers.* Rochestor, VT: Bear & Company.

Melson, G. F. (2000). Companion animals and the development of children: Implications of the biophilia hypothesis. In A. Fine (Ed.), *Handbook on Animal-Assisted Therapy: Theoretical Foundations and Guidelines for Practice* (pp. 375–383). San Diego, CA: Academic Press.

Melson, G. F. (2001). *Why the Wild Things Are: Animals in the Lives of Children.* Cambridge, MA: Harvard University Press.

Melson, G. F., and Fine, A. H. (2006). Animals in the lives of children. In A. H. Fine (Ed.), *Handbook on Animal-Assisted Therapy: Theoretical Foundations and Guidelines for Practice* (2nd ed.) (pp. 207–226). San Diego, CA: Academic Press.

Melson, G. F., Schwarz, R., and Beck, A. M. (1998). *Pets as Sources of Support for Mothers, Fathers, and Young Children.* Paper presented to the Eight International Conference in Human-Animal Interaction, Prague.

Messent, P. R. (1983). Social facilitation of contact with other people by pet dogs. In A. H. Katcher and A. M. Beck (Eds.), *New Perspectives on Our Lives With Companion Animals* (pp. 37–46). Philadelphia: University of Philadelphia Press.

Messent, P. R., and Serpell, J. A. (1981). A historical and biological view of the pet owner bond. In B. Fogle (Ed.), *Interrelations Between People and Pets* (pp. 5–22). Springfield, IL: Charles C Thomas.

Miller, J. (2000). Perioperative nursing and animal-assisted therapy [Online]. *Association of Operating Room Nurses, Inc.* Retrieved May 20, 2003. Available: http://www.findarticles.com/cf_0/m0FSL/3_72/ 65539098/print.jhtml

Morse, J., and Field, P. (1995). *Qualitative Research Methods for Health Professionals* (2nd ed.). Thousand Oaks, CA: Sage Publications.

Morse, J., and Richards, L. (2002). *Read Me First For a User's Guide to Qualitative Methods.* Thousand Oaks, CA: Sage Publications.

Moustakas, C. (1994). *Phenomenological Research Methods.* Thousand Oaks, CA: Sage Publications.

Mugford, R., and McComisky, J. (1975). Some recent work on the psychotherapeutic value of cage birds with old people. In R. S. Anderson (Ed.), *Pet Animals and Society* (pp. 54–65). London: Baillere Tindall.

Muschel, I. (1984). Pet therapy with terminal cancer patients. *Social Casework, 65,* 451–458.

Muschel, I. (1985). Pet therapy with terminal cancer patients. *The Latham Letter,* fall, 8–15.

Musil, R. (1970). Domestication of the dog already in the Magdalenian? *Anthropologies, 8,* 87–88.

Najavitis, L. M., and Strupp, H. H. (1994). Differences in effectiveness of psychodynamic therapists: A process-outcome study. *Psychotherapy, 31,* 187–197.

Newby, J. (1999). *The Animal Attraction: Humans and Their Animal Companions.* Sydney, NSW: ABC Books.

Nicoll, K. (2005). *Soul Friends: Finding Healing with Animals.* Indianapolis, IN: Dog Ear Publishing.

Nightingale, F. (1859). *Notes on Nursing: What is and What is Not.* London, England: Harrison & Sons.

Noonan, E. (1998). People and pets. *Psychodynamic Counselling, 4,* 17–31.

Nouwen, H. (1979). *The Wounded Healer: Ministry in Contemporary Society.* New York: Doubleday.

Olsen, S. J., and Olsen, J. W. (1977). The Chinese world ancestor of new world dogs. *Science, 197,* 533–535.

Palmatier, R. A. (1995). *Speaking of Animals: A Dictionary of Animal Metaphors.* Westport, CT: Greenwood Press.

Parshall, D. P. (2003). Research and reflection: Animal-assisted therapy in mental health settings. *Counseling and Values, 48*, 47–56.

Patton, M. Q. (2002). *Qualitative Research & Evaluation Methods.* Thousand Oaks, CA: Sage Publications.

Patronek, G. J., and Glickman, L. T. (1993). Pet ownership protects the risks and consequences of coronary heart disease. *Medical Hypotheses, 40*, 245–349.

Perin, C. (1981). Dogs as symbols in human development. In B. Fogle (Ed.), *Interrelations Between People and Pets* (pp. 68–88). Springfield, IL: Charles C Thomas.

Pine, F. (1984). The interpretive moment. *Bulletin of the Menninger Clinic, 48*, 54–71.

Phillips, A. (1988). *Winnicott.* Cambridge, MA: Harvard University Press.

Randour, M. L. (2000). *Animal Grace: Entering a Spiritual Relationship with Our Fellow Creatures.* Novato, CA: New World Library.

Reichert, E. (1998). Individual counseling for sexually abused children: A role for animals and storytelling. *Child and Adolescent Social Work Journal, 15*, 177–185.

Rivas, J., and Burghardt, G. M. (2002). Crotalomorphism: A metaphor for understanding anthropomorphism by omission. In M. Bekoff, C. Allen, and G. M. Burghardt (Eds.), *The Cognitive Animal: Empirical and Theoretical Perspectives on Animal Cognition* (pp. 9–17). Cambridge, MA: Bradford Books.

Robbins, A. (1987). An object relations approach to art therapy. In J. A. Rubin (Ed.), *Approaches to Art Therapy,* (pp. 63–74). New York: Brunner-Routledge.

Robin, M., tenBensel, R. W., Quingly, J. S., and Anderson, R. K. (1983). Childhood pets and psychosocial development of adolescence. In A. H. Katcher, and A. M. Beck (Eds.), *New Perspectives in Our Lives with Companion Animals* (pp. 436–443). Philadelphia: University of Pennsylvania Press.

Robinson, D., and Reed, V. (Eds.). (1998). *The A-Z of Social Research Jargon.* Aldershot, UK: Ashgate.

Rogers, C. (1951). *Client-Centered Therapy.* Boston: Houghton Mifflin.

Rogers, C. (1961). *On Becoming a Person: A Therapist's View of Psychotherapy.* Boston: Houghton Mifflin.

Rogers, C. (1989). *On Becoming a Person.* New York: Houghton Mifflin.

Rossbach, K. A., and Wilson, J. P. (1992). Does a dog's presence make a person appear more likeable? *Anthrozoos, 5*, 40–51.

Rost, D. H., and Hartmann, A. (1994). Children and their pets. *Anthrozoos, 7*, 242–254.

Rousell, J. O. (1999). *Dealing with Grief, Theirs and Ours.* New York: Alba House.

Rowan, A. N., and Thayer, L. (2000). Forward. In A. H. Fine (Ed.), *Handbook on Animal-Assisted Therapy: Theoretical Foundations and Guidlines for Practice* (pp. xxvii–xliv). New York: Academic Press.

Ruckert, J. (1987). *The Four-Footed Therapist: How Your Pet Can Help You Solve Your Problems.* Berkeley, CA: Ten Speed Press.

Rynearson, E. K. (1978). Humans and pets and attachment. *British Journal of Psychiatry, 133*, 550–555.

Sable, P. (1995). Pets, attachment, and well-being across the life cycle. *Social Work, 40*, 334–341.

Sadala, M., and Adorno, R. (2002). Phenomenology as a method to investigate the experience lived: A perspective from Husserl and Merleau Ponty's thought. *Journal of Advanced Nursing, 37*, 282–293.

Sams, J., and Carson. D. (1999). *Medicine Cards*. New York: St. Martin's Press.

Sarmicanic, L. (2004). Goffman, pets, and people: An analysis of humans and their companion animals. *ReVision, 27*, 42–47.

Scharff, J. S., and Scharff, D. E. (1995). *The Primer of Object Relations Theory*. Lanham, MD: The Rowman & Littlefield Publishing Group, Inc.

Schoen, A. M. (2001). *Kindred Spirits: How the Remarkable Bond Between Humans and Animals Can Change the Way We Live*. New York: Random House, Inc

Schoen, A. M., and Proctor, P. (1995). *Love, Miracles, and Animal Healing: A Heart Warming Look at the Spiritual Bond Between Animals and Humans*. New York: Fireside.

Seamon, D. (2000). *Phenomenology, place environment and architecture: A review of literature* [Online]. Retrieved January 15, 2005. Available: http://www.arch.ksu.edu/ seamon/articles/2000_phenomenology_ review.htm

Seinfeld, J. (1993). *Interpreting and Holding: The Paternal and Maternal Functions of the Psychotherapist*. Northvale, New Jersey: Jason Aronson Inc.

Serpell, J. A. (1991). Beneficial effects of pet ownership on some aspects of human health and behaviour. *Journal of the Royal Society of Medicine, 84*, 717–720.

Serpell, J. A. (1993). Animals in children's lives [Online]. *Society & Animals, 1*. Retrieved September 23, 2005. Available: http://www .psyeta.org//sa/sa7.2/serpell.html

Serpell, J. A. (2000a). Animal companions and human well-being: An historical exploration of the value of human-animal relationships. In A. H. Fine (Ed.), *Handbook on Animal-Assisted Therapy* (pp. 3–19). New York: Academic Press.

Serpell, J. A. (2000b). Creatures of the unconscious: Companion animals as mediators. In A. L. Podberscek, E. S. Paul, and J. A. Serpell (Eds.). *Companion Animals & Us: Exploring the Relationships Between People and Pets* (pp. 108–121). New York: Cambridge University Press.

Serpell, J. A. (2006). Animal-assisted interventions in historical perspective. In A. H. Fine (Ed.), *Handbook on Animal-Assisted Therapy: Theoretical Foundations and Guidelines for Practice* (2nd ed.) (pp. 3–20). San Diego, CA: Academic Press.

Serpell, J. A., Coppinger, R., and Fine, A. H. (2006). Welfare considerations in therapy and assistance dogs. In A. H. Fine (Ed.), *Handbook on Animal-Assisted Therapy: Theoretical Foundations and Guidelines for Practice* (2nd ed.), (pp. 453-474). San Diego, CA: Academic Press.

Serpell, J., and Paul, E. (1994). Pets and the development of positive attitudes to animals. In A. Manning and J. Serpell (Eds.), *Animals and Human Society: Changing Perspectives* (pp. 127–144). London: Routledge.

Sherbourne, C. D., Meredith, L. S., Rogers, W., and Ware, J. E. (1992). Social support and stressful life events: Age differences in their effects on health-related quality of life among the chronically ill. *Quality of Life Research, 1*, 235–246.

Shiloh, S., Sorek, G., and Terkel, J. (2003). Reduction of state-anxiety by petting animals in a controlled laboratory experiment. A*nxiety, Stress, and Coping, 16*, 387–395.

Bibliography 151

Siegal, A. (1962). Reaching the severely withdrawn through pet therapy. *American Journal of Psychiatry, 118*, 1045–1046.

Siegel, J. M. (1990). Stressful life events and use of physician services among the elderly: The moderating role of pet ownership. *Journal of Personality and Social Psychology, 58*, 1081–1086.

Simington, J. (1996). The response of the human spirit to loss. *Living With Our Losses Bereavement Magazine, 1*, 9–11.

Simington, J. (2003). *Journey to the Sacred: Mending a Fractured Soul.* Edmonton: Taking Flight.

Simington, J. (2005). *Responding Soul to Soul: During Times of Spiritual Uprooting.* Edmonton, AB: Taking Flight.

Simington, J., and Victorian Order of Nurses (1999). *Listening to soul pain.* (Audio visual). Edmonton, AB: Souleado Productions.

Slochower, J. (1996). *Holding and Psychoanalysis: A Relational Perspective.* Mahwah, NJ: The Analytic Press.

Schmitt, R. (1967). Husserl's trancendental-phenomenological reduction. In J. J. Kockelmans (Ed.), *Phenomenology* (pp. 58–68) Garden City, NY: Doubleday.

Spitz, R. (1946). Hospitalism. *The Psychoanalytic Study of the Child, II*, 113–117.

Staker, C., Watson, D., & Robinson, T. (2002). Trauma and disconnection: A trans-theoretical approach. *International Journal of Psychotherapy, 7*, 145–158.

Stone, C. (2002). *The Incidental Guru: Lessons in Healing from a Dog.* Markham, Ontario; Fitzhenry & Whiteside.

Strand, E. B. (2004). Interparental conflict and youth maladjustment: The Buffering effects of pets. *Stress, Trauma, and Crisis, 7*, 151–168.

Taylor, C. W. (1991). *The Skilled Pastor: Counseling as the Practice of Theology.* Minneapolis: Fortress Press.

Triebenbacher, S. L. (1998). Pets as transitional objects: Their role in children's emotional development. *Psychological Reports, 82*, 191–200.

Truax, C. B., and Carkhuff, R. R. (1967). *Toward effective counselling and psychotherapy: Training and practice.* Chicago: Aldine-Atherton.

Turner, D. C. (2000). The role of ethology in the field of human-animal relations and animal-assisted therapy. In A. Fine (Ed.) *Handbook on Animal-Assisted Therapy: Theoretical Foundations and Guidelines for Practice* (pp. 449–459). San Diego, CA: Academic Press.

Ubelacker, S. (2005, Sept. 12). Pets stranded by Katrina wrench hearts. *Edmonton Journal*, p. A2.

Ulrich, R. S. (1984). View through a window may influence recovery from surgery. *Science, 224*, 420–421.

Urichuk, L., and Anderson, D. (2003). *Improving Mental Health Through Animal-Assisted Therapy.* Edmonton, AB: The Chimo Project.

Van Manen, M. (1997). *Researching Lived Experience* (2nd ed.). London, Ontario: Althouse Press.

Vilhajamson, R. (1993). Life stress, social support and clinical depression: A reanalysis of the literature. *Social Science Medicine, 37*, 331–342.

Wells, E. S., Rosen, L. W., and Walshaw, S. (1997). Use of feral cats in psychotherapy. *Anthrozoos 10*, 125–130.

Welman, J. C., and Kruger, S. J. (1999). *Research Methodology for the Business and Administrative Sciences.* Johannesburg, South Africa: Oxford University Press.

Wilber, K. (1998). *The Essential Ken Wilber: An Introductory Reader.* Boston: Shambhala Publications, Inc.

Wilson, C. C. (2006). Human-Animal Interactions and Health: Best Evidence and Where We Go From Here. In A.H. Fine (Ed.) *Handbook on animal-assisted therapy: theoretical foundations and guidelines for practice* (2nd ed.), (pp. 499–512). San Diego, CA: Academic Press.

Wilson, E. O. (1984). *Biophilia.* Cambridge, MA: Harvard University Press.

Wilson, E. O. (1993). Biophilia and the conservation ethic. In S. R. Kellert & E. O. Wilson (Eds.), *The Bbiophilia Hypothesis* (pp. 31–41). Washington, DC: Island Press/Shearwater Books.

Wilson, L. M. (1972). Intensive care delirium: The effect of outside deprivation in a windowless unit. *Archives of Internal Medicine, 130*, 123–145.

Winnicott, D. W. (1958). Mind and its relation to the psyche-soma. In D. W. Winnicott(1958), *Through Pediatrics to Psycho-Analysis*, (pp. 243–254). New York: Basic Books.

Winnicott, D. W. (2005). Transitional objects and transitional phenomena. In D. W. Winnicott, *Playing and reality* (pp. 1–34). New York: Routledge.

Winnicott, D. W. (1965). The capacity to be alone. In D. W. Winnicott, *The Maturational Processes and the Facilitating Environment* (pp. 29–36). New York: International Universities Press.

Winnicott, D. W. (1965). The aims of psychoanalytic treatment. In D. Winnicott, *The Maturational Processes and the Facilitating Environment* (pp. 166–170). New York: International Universities Press.

Winnicott, D. W. (1964). *The Family and Individual Development.* London: Tavistock.

Winnicott, D. W. (1965). *The Maturational Processes and the Facilitating Environment.* New YorkY: International Press.

Winnicott, D. W. (1971/2005). *Playing and reality.* New York: Routledge.

Winnicott, D. W. (1987). *Home is Where We Start from: Essays by a Psychoanalyst.* London: Pelican Books.

Wishon, P. (1989). Disease and injury from companion animals. *Early Child Development and Care, 46*, 31–38.

Woloy, E. (1990). *The Symbol of the Dog in the Human Psyche: A Study of the Human Dog Bond.* Wilmette, IL.: Chiron Publications.

Wood, M. W. (2006). Techniques for searching the animal-assisted therapy literature. In A. H. Fine (Ed.), *Handbook on Animal-Assisted Therapy: Theoretical Foundations and Guidelines for Practice* (2nd ed.), (pp. 413–424). San Diego, CA: Academic Press.

Wyatt-Brown, A. M. (1993). From the clinic to the classroom: D. W. Winnicott, James Britton, and the revolution in writing theory. In P. L. Rudnytsky, *Transitional Objects and Potential Spaces: Literary Uses of D. W. Winnicott* (pp. 292–305). New York: Columbia University Press.

Zeuner, F. E. (1963). *A History of Domesticated Animals.* New York: Harper & Row.

INDEX

A

AAA (*see* Animal-assisted activity)
AAT (*see* Animal-assisted therapy)
Acceptance
    in therapeutic environment, 81–82
    unconditional, 136
Adjunct therapy
    in professional practice, 84–85
    as theme, 133
Agape, 88, 117
Agreements
    audiotaping, 124
    interview, 121–122
Alliance/relationship, therapeutic
    enhanced healing, catalyst for, 80
    enhancing, 98–100
    as theme, 79–80, 132
    trust, 79–80
Animal-assisted activity (AAA), 35–36, 117
Animal-assisted interventions, 36, 117
Animal-assisted therapy (AAT)
    defined, 35–36, 117
    history, 13–14, 31–36
    and holding environment, 104–105
    matching clients, 107–108
    and mentally ill, 32–35
    and trauma, 36–37, 100–104
        future research, 106–107
    and work environment, 108
    see also Companion animals
Animal selection, 110
Animal welfare, 109–110
Attachment behavior, 7

B

Bethel (Germany), 32–33

Biophilia Hypothesis
    and the Christian Bible, 23–25
    drawbacks, 24
    and human health, 22–23
    see also Wilson, E. O.
Bowlby, J., 7
Bracketing, 50, 52

C

Cats
    as companion animals, 15–16
    domestication, 19–20
    see also Companion animals
Chimo Project (Canada), 42–43, 45, 118
Christianity, 23–25
    see also Religion
Clients, selection
    and animal-assisted therapy, 107–108
    ethical considerations, 111–112
Columbine High School (1999), 103, 107
Companion animals
    defined, 118
    and dissociation, 36
    domestication, 19–21
    other animals, 107–108
    vs. "pet," 20–21, 119
    and trauma, 36–37
    and work environment, 104
    see also Animal-assisted therapy
Confidentiality
    ethical considerations, 41–42
    judge, independent, 128
    transcriber, 127
Constriction, 101–102
    see also Trauma
Counseling (*see* Professional practice)
Creativity

153

environment, enhanced therapeutic, 83
as theme, 136

D

Delta Society, 26, 35, 87, 118
Dissociation, 36–37, 102–103
    see also Trauma
Dogs
    domestication, 19–20
    and historical leaders, 31
    as "ice breakers," 29–30
    and mother love, 16
    nature of, 8
    see also Companion animals

E

Environment
    holding (*see* Holding environment)
    therapeutic
        acceptance, unconditional, 81–82
        creativity, 83
        enhanced, 80–83, 133, 135
        enhancing, 98–100
        nurture, 82–83
        safety, 80–81, 135
    work, 104
Ethical considerations
    animal welfare, 109–110
    confidentiality, 41–42
    responsibility, 42
    selection
        animal, 110
        client, 111–112
    see also Confidentiality; Professional practice

F

Freud, Sigmund, 31–32

G

Glossary, 117–120
"Good-enough-mother," 118
    see also Transitional phenomena

H

Hall, Granville Stanley, 21

Healing, enhanced
    as theme, 135
    in therapeutic alliance/relationship, 80
Holding environment
    defined, 119
    summary, 96
    themes, application of, 79–89
    and transitional phenomena, 77–79
    see also Environment
Human-animal bond
    history, 26–27
    and human health, 28
    professionals, interest of, 27–28
    research, 26–28
    and social theory, 29–30
Hurricane Katrina (2005), 3
Hyperarousal, 9, 101
    see also Trauma

I

Information collection
    methods, 49–51
        interviews, 49–50
        storing data, 51
    participants, 42–43
        interviews, 45–49
        selection, 43–45
    trustworthiness, 55
    see also Interviews
Interviews
    agreement, 122–123
    analysis and interpretation, 51–54
    audiorecordings, 50–51
    bracketing, 52
    checklist, 121
    meaning, units of
        clustering, 52–53
        delineating, 52
    modifying, 53–54
    participants, 45–49
    questions, 38–39
    reduction, phenomenological, 52
    return to the participant, 53–54
    summarizing, 53–54
        composite, 54
    themes, 52–54
        contextualization, 54
    validating, 53
    see also Information collection;
        Participants

Index

Intrusion, 101
    see also Trauma

J

Judges, independent, 42, 55, 128

L

Levinson, Boris, 26, 33–34, 106
Loneliness, 29

M

Meaning, units of
    clustering, 52, 130–131
    delineating, 52, 129
Methods, 39–41

N

Nightingale, Florence, 32
Nurture
    environment, enhanced therapeutic, 82–83
    as theme, 136

O

Object relations theory, 76–77, 91, 116
Objects, transitional (*see* Transitional objects)
Oklahoma City bombing (1995), 106

P

Participants
    demographics, 125–126
    interviews, 45–49
    selection, 43–45
    see also Interviews
Pawling Army Air Corps Convalescent Hospital
    (New York), 33
Phenomenology
    defined, 40–41
    reduction, 52
    transcendental, 40
Potential space (*see* Transitional space)
Professional practice
    enhanced, 84–86
        adjunct therapy, 84–85

    as theme, 136
ethical considerations, 108–112
    animal selection, 110
    animal welfare, 109–110
    client selection, 111–112
future research, 104–108
    other frameworks, 105–106
implications, 98–104
as theme, 134
Project, basis for, 39

R

Reduction, phenomenological, 52
Religion
    and the Biophilia Hypothesis, 23–25
    sacredness, sense of, 86–89
    spirituality, 103

S

Sacredness
    sense of, 86–89, 95
    as theme, 133, 136–137
    see also Religion
Space, transitional (*see* Transitional space)
Spirituality, 103
    see also Religion
Support theory, 29–30

T

Taylor, Charles W., 81
Themes
    alliance/relationship, therapeutic, 79–80,
    132, 135
    basic, 132–134
    final, 135–137
    holding environment, 79–89
    interviews, 52–54
        contextualization, 54
    transitional phenomena, 89–94
Therapy (*see* Animal-assisted therapy)
Thurston High School (1998), 107
Transcribers, 124
"Transitional beings," 93, 120
Transitional objects
    animals as, 10
    defined, 78, 92, 120

themes, application of, 92–94
Transitional phenomena
    defined, 78
    and holding environment, 77–79
    objects (transitional), 92–94
    relationship, 120
    space (transitional), 89–92
    summary, 97
    themes, application of, 89–94
    see also Transitional object; Transitional
       space
Transitional space
    defined, 78, 89, 120
    themes, application of, 89–92
Trauma
    and animal-assisted therapy, 100–104
    and dissociation, 36–37
    and hyperarousal, 9
Trust, 79–80, 135

W

Welfare (*see* Animal welfare)
Well-being (of therapist), 85–86, 133
Wilson, E. O., 21–22
    see also Biophilia Hypothesis
Winnicott, D. W.
    developmental theory, vii, 6, 10–12, 83
    holding environment, 77–79
    themes, application of, 79–94
    transitional phenomena, 77–79
    Work environment (*see* Environment)
    World Trade Center (2001), 106

Y

York Retreat (England), 32

Charles C Thomas
PUBLISHER • LTD.

P.O. Box 19265
Springfield, IL 62794-9265

- Bellini, James L. & Phillip D. Rumrill, Jr.—**RESEARCH IN REHABILITATION COUNSELING: A Guide to Design, Methodology, and Utilization. (2nd Ed.)** '09, 318 pp. (7 x 10) 3 il., 5 tables.

- Brooke, Stephanie L.—**THE USE OF THE CREATIVE THERAPIES WITH CHEMICAL DEPENDECY ISSUES.** '09, 300 pp. (7 x 10), 33 il., 3 tables.

- Johnson, David Read & Renee Emunah—**CURRENT APPROACHES IN DRAMA THERAPY. (2nd Ed.)** '09, (7 x 10) 11 il.

- Luginbuehl-Oelhafen, Ruth R.—**ART THERAPY WITH CHRONIC PHYSICALLY ILL ADOLESCENTS: Exploring the Effectiveness of Medical Art Therapy as a Complementary Treatment.** '09, 220 pp. (7 x 10), 67 il., (12 in color), $37.95, paper.

- McNiff, Shaun—**INTEGRATING THE ARTS IN THERAPY: History, Theory, and Practice.** '09, 272 pp. (7 x 10), 60 il.

- Wilkes, Jane K.—**THE ROLE OF COMPANION ANIMALS IN COUNSELING AND PSYCHOTHERAPY: Discovering Their Use in the Therapeutic Process.** '09,172 pp. (7 x 10), 2 tables, paper.

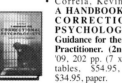

- Correia, Kevin M.—**A HANDBOOK FOR CORRECTIONAL PSYCHOLOGISTS: Guidance for the Prison Practitioner. (2nd Ed.)** '09, 202 pp. (7 x 10), 3 tables, $54.95, hard, $34.95, paper.

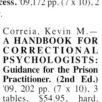

- Horovitz, Ellen G. & Sarah L. Eksten—**THE ART THERAPISTS' PRIMER: A Clinical Guide to Writing Assessments, Diagnosis, & Treatment.** '09, 332 pp. (7 x 10), 106 il., 2 tables, $85.95, hard, $55.95, paper.

- Kocsis, Richard N.—**APPLIED CRIMINAL PSYCHOLOGY: A Guide to Forensic Behavioral Sciences.** '09, 306 pp. (7 x 10), 4 il., 2 tables, $65.95, hard, $45.95, paper.

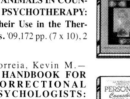

- Moon, Bruce L.—**EXISTENTIAL ART THERAPY: The Canvas Mirror. (3rd Ed.)** '09, 284 pp. (7 x 10), 51 il., $64.95, hard, $44.95, paper.

- Richard, Michael A., William G. Emener, & William S. Hutchison, Jr.—**EMPLOYEE ASSISTANCE PROGRAMS: Wellness/Enhancement Programming. (4th Ed.)** '09, 428 pp. (8 x 10), 8 il., 1 table, $79.95, hard, $57.95, paper.

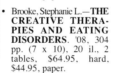

- Brooke, Stephanie L.—**THE CREATIVE THERAPIES AND EATING DISORDERS.** '08, 304 pp. (7 x 10), 20 il., 2 tables, $64.95, hard, $44.95, paper.

- Geldard, Kathryn & David Geldard—**PERSONAL COUNSELING SKILLS: An Integrative Approach.** '08, 316 pp. (7 x 10), 20 il., 3 tables, $49.95, paper.

- Junge, Maxine Borowsky—**MOURNING, MEMORY AND LIFE ITSELF: Essays by an Art Therapist.** '08, 292 pp. (7 x 10), 38 il, $61.95, hard, $41.95, paper.

- Kendler, Howard H.—**AMORAL THOUGHTS ABOUT MORALITY: The Intersection of Science, Psychology, and Ethics. (2nd Ed.)** '08, 270 pp. (7 x 10), $59.95, hard, $39.95, paper.

- Wiseman, Dennis G.—**THE AMERICAN FAMILY: Understanding its Changing Dynamics and Place in Society.** '08, 172 pp. (7 x 10), 4 tables, $31.95, paper.

- Arrington, Doris Banowsky—**ART, ANGST, AND TRAUMA: Right Brain Interventions with Developmental Issues.** '07, 278 pp. (7 x 10), 123 il., (10 in color, paper edition only), $63.95, hard, $48.95, paper.

- Daniels, Thomas & Allen Ivey—**MICROCOUNSELING: Making Skills Training Work In a Multicultural World.** '07, 296 pp. (7 x 10), 12 il., 3 tables, $65.95, hard, $45.95, paper.

- Olson, R. Paul—**MENTAL HEALTH SYSTEMS COMPARED: Great Britain, Norway, Canada, and the United States.** '06, 398 pp. (8 1/2 x 11), 10 il., 65 tables, $89.95, hard, $64.95, paper.

5 easy ways to order!

PHONE: 1-800-258-8980 or (217) 789-8980

FAX: (217) 789-9130

EMAIL: books@ccthomas.com
Web: www.ccthomas.com

MAIL: Charles C Thomas • Publisher, Ltd.
P.O. Box 19265
Springfield, IL 62794-9265

Complete catalog available at ccthomas.com • books@ccthomas.com

Books sent on approval • Shipping charges: $7.75 min. U.S. / Outside U.S., actual shipping fees will be charged • Prices subject to change without notice